1000 INTRODUCTORY TOXICOLOGY REVIEW QUESTIONS

1000 INTRODUCTORY TOXICOLOGY REVIEW QUESTIONS

Richard Fruncillo MD PhD

ISBN: 1544224346
ISBN 13: 9781544224343
Library of Congress Control Number: 2017915571
CreateSpace Independent Publishing Platform
North Charleston, South Carolina

Contents

Disclaimer

The clinical questions in this review book were chosen from some of the most recent and well-respected textbooks in the field. However, it is well-known that the standard of care in the practice of medicine can change rapidly. Every week, hundreds of clinically relevant new scientific journal articles are published worldwide. I am old enough to remember many examples of drugs that were indicated in the treatment of the certain disease at the beginning of my career, that later became contraindicated. While I have made great efforts to ensure the accuracy of the information in this book at the time of publication, the possibility of human error still exists. Neither the author nor the publisher can guarantee that the information contained in this book is complete and accurate, and both disclaim any responsibility for any inaccuracies. Therefore, anyone using the clinical information contained in this book for direct patient care must absolutely confirm that it is still within the standard of care in their community. It is particularly important to check drug dosages, indications, interactions, and contraindications with the manufacturer's most recent product information. Also, the information in this book should not be interpreted by non-physician readers as advice for the treatment of drug overdose. Discussions with major Poison Control Centers are strongly recommend. Neither the author nor the publisher will assume liability for damages that result from use of the information contained in any part of this book.

Preface

The purpose of this book is to learn toxicology. The information sources for these questions have come from many of the most recent introductory textbooks in the area. I remember from my medical school days, that the best way to comprehend the overwhelming amount of material presented was repetition in different formats. You needed to hear it in the classroom and on rounds, see it in texts, and as I found to be one of the most productive ways, review test questions. Until this day, I rarely forgot a piece of information that I answered incorrectly on a test and later looked up. I have tried to emphasize principles. I have made every attempt only have one best answer to each question. However, in a book of 1000 questions, there may be a few that are ambiguous or repetitious. This book should be useful to those taking their first course in general toxicology.

1

General Principles

1. The basic principle of toxicology is ___.

    A. the dose makes the poison

    B. every poison has an antidote

    C. one man's poison is another man's vitamin

    D. if something is toxic to lab animals, it must be toxic to humans

2. The founder of modern toxicology was___.

    A. Archimedes

    B. Euclid

    C. Paracelsus

    D. Pythagoras

3. The difference between a toxin and a toxicant is ___.

    A. a toxin has an antidote

    B. a toxicant is a protein

    C. a toxin is of biological origin

    D. A toxicant has a U -shaped dose response curve

4. Which of the following statements is/are true?

    A. natural products are always safer than man-made chemicals

    B. over-the-counter dietary supplements are evaluated by the FDA in the same manner as prescription drugs

    C. both

    D. neither

5. The most common type of quantal dose-response curve is ___.

    A. U shaped

    B. inverted U-shaped

    C. a sine wave

    D. somewhat similar to an S

6. All the following are true regarding the reasons why a toxicant affects a target organ except ___.

    A. the toxicant may be present there in high concentration

    B. a toxic metabolite may be produced in the organ

    C. the organ may contain high concentrations of vitamin C which is synergistic with the toxicant

    D. special transporters may bring the toxicant into the organ cells

7. In toxicology, a target organ is considered ___.

    A. an organ demonstrating a major toxic effect from the toxicant
    B. the organ with the highest concentration of toxicant
    C. the organ that is first exposed to the toxicant
    D the organ that most resists the toxic effects of the toxicant

8. When the sum of two toxic effects is greater than the sum of the individual effects, the result is called ___.

    A. synergy
    B. additivity
    C. geometric progression
    D. compound toxicity

9. A toxicant that is absorbed through the gastrointestinal tract and subsequently affects the brain and nervous system, is said to have a/an ___.

    A. chronic effect
    B. systemic effect
    C. local effect
    D. reversible effect

10. Liver cirrhosis present years after discontinuing alcohol use is considered a/an ___.

    A. irreversible effect
    B. allergic reaction
    C. both
    D. neither

11. If a toxicant binds to a part of a cell, and the interaction initiates a physical or chemical signal uy7to the cell, the process is called ___.

    A. initiation
    B. toxicant – receptor interaction
    C. cell to cell communication
    D. apoptosis

12. The octanol/water partition coefficient of a chemical is a measure of ___.

    A. acid pH
    B. basic pH
    C. free energy
    D. lipid solubility

13. In certain individuals, a U shaped graded dose – toxic response curve will be produced by ___.

A. lead
B. botulinum toxin
C. vitamins
D. anthrax

14. All the following bind to human receptors to exert their pharmacologic effect except ___.

A. dopamine
B. epinephrine
C. acetylcholine
D. tetrafluoromethane

15. A molecule that binds to a physiologic receptor is called a ___.

A. ligand
B. coordination compound
C. resonance molecule
D. reagent

16. A carrier that transports chemicals out of cells is ___.

A. albumin
B. P-glycoprotein
C. Gamma – globulin
D. orosomucoid

17. A rare, genetically related, non-– dose – related reaction to a drug or chemical is called a/an ___.

    A. hypersensitivity reaction
    B. mutagenic reaction
    C. idiosyncratic reaction
    D. Grignard reaction

18. A molecule that binds to a receptor but has no activity at the receptor is called a/an ___.

    A. negative ligand
    B. antagonist
    C. partial agonist
    D. zero binder

19. A molecule that is dosed at the NOAEL in rats ___.

    A. will be toxic 50% of the time in the rat
    B. will be safe in every other type of laboratory animal
    C. will be lethal to 10% of rats
    D. should not demonstrate any observable adverse effects in the rat

20. Which of the following is least likely to be involved in a toxic response if it toxicant binds to it?

    A. enzyme
    B. DNA
    C. extracellular structural protein
    D. cell membrane

21. LD50 is a measure of ___.

    A. chronic toxicity
    B. cancer-causing potential
    C. acute toxicity
    D. allergy potential

22. A person concerned with the treatment of a victim of drug overdose is a ___.

    A. descriptive toxicologist
    B. forensic toxicologist
    C. regulatory toxicologist
    D. clinical toxicologist

23. Which of the following is not a type of toxicologist?

    A. mechanistic toxicologist
    B. reproductive toxicologist
    C. anatomic toxicologist
    D. environmental toxicologist

24. Haptens ___.

    A. form DNA adducts

    B. combine with a protein to form an antigen

    C. combine with lipids to create pores in cell membranes

    D. block the allergic response

25. When a non-toxic chemical makes another chemical more toxic, the result is called ___.

    A. synergism

    B. potentiation

    C. multiplication

    D. exponential effect

26. The highest dose point on the graded dose-response curve in which no adverse effects are seen is called the ___.

    A. starting point

    B. NOAEL

    C. margin of safety

    D. safety threshold

27. An immune – mediated toxic effect that occurs after a previous exposure to a chemical is called ___.

    A. irritant response

    B. allergic response

    C. inflammatory response

    D. counterregulatory response

28. Significant exposure to a toxicant can occur by ___.

    A. oral ingestion
    B. skin exposure
    C. inhalation
    D. all the above

29. When performing toxicology tests on laboratory animals to help understand toxic effects in humans, ___.

    A. high doses of toxicants are used
    B. at least 1000 animals must be tested
    C. only male animals are used
    D. only nonhuman primates are used

30. Toxicity testing is performed animals to ___.

    A. unequivocally prove that a chemical is safe in humans
    B. understand the toxic effects the chemical can produce
    C. both
    D. neither

31. Toxicity testing in animals involves ___.

    A. analysis of blood for biochemical abnormalities
    B. organ tissue examination for abnormalities
    C. both
    D. neither

32. If the LD50 is 25 mg/kg in a mouse, and 50 mg/kg in a rat, which of the following statements is/are true?

  A. the chemical is acutely more toxic in the mouse then in the rat
  B. 20 mg/kg is a safe dose for humans
  C. the LD50 in any rodent cannot be greater than 100 mg/kg
  D. all the above

33. Which of the following statements is true regarding the LD50?

  A. It only measures acute lethality.
  B. It must be normalized to the surface area of the animal.
  C. both
  D. neither

34. *In vitro* testing means ___.

  A. performing tests on live laboratory animals
  B. performing tests without the use of live laboratory animals
  C. performing tests on bacteria and protozoa only
  D. performing tests on plants and fungi only

35. *In vivo* testing means ___.

  A. performing tests on live laboratory animals
  B. performing tests without the use of live laboratory animals
  C. performing tests on bacteria and protozoa only
  D. performing tests on plant and fungi only

36. LC 50 represents ___.

    A. the concentration of toxicant at the LD50

    B. the concentration of toxicant in air or water that kills 50% of the animals over a specified time

    C. the lowest concentration of toxicant that kills 50% of the animals in 10 different animal species

    D. none of the above

37. Genetic polymorphisms ___.

    A. are due solely to chromosomal aneuploidy

    B. cause differences in response to a toxicant in the same species

    C. both

    D. neither

38. Which of the following quantal dose-response curves represents the safest type of toxicant?

    A. a steep dose- response curve

    B. a dose-response curve without a threshold

    C. a somewhat flat dose-response curve

    D. a vertical dose-response curve

39. Acute exposure to a toxicant involves ___?

    A. a single exposure

    B. exposure by inhalation for less than 24 hours

    C. both

    D. neither

40. A state of decreased receptor response to the effect of a toxicant after repeated exposure is called ___.

    A. resistance
    B. acquiescence
    C. tolerance
    D. reverse toxicity

41. When the sum of the toxic effects of two chemicals is equal to the sum of their individual toxic effects the result is called ___.

    A. synergy
    B. additivity
    C. potentiation
    D. agonism

42. The type of toxicologist who establishes standards for the concentrations of chemicals allowed in foods, air, and drinking water is called a ___.

    A. mechanistic toxicologist
    B. developmental toxicologist
    C. medical toxicologist
    D. regulatory toxicologist

43. The type of toxicologist that studies adverse effects on an embryo, fetus, or newborn that results from exposure to toxicants at the time of conception or during gestation is called a ___.

    A. descriptive toxicologist
    B. developmental toxicologist
    C. mechanistic toxicologist
    D. medical toxicologist

44. The type of toxicologist that is involved with medical- legal aspects of toxicology is called a___.

    A. descriptive toxicologist
    B. medical toxicologist
    C. legal toxicologist
    D. forensic toxicologist

45. Which of the following statements is true?

    A. The liver is a very infrequent target organ for toxicity.
    B. The pancreas is a very frequent target organ for toxicity.
    C. both
    D. neither

46. The dose on a dose-response curve is frequently plotted in ___.

    A. base 10 logarithmic units
    B. base e logarithmic units
    C. milligrams per liter of organism volume
    D. all the above

47. Animals demonstrating toxicity at the left end of a quantal dose-response curve are referred to as ___.

A resistant
B allergic
C hyper-susceptible
B hyposensitive

48. Animals exhibiting toxicity at the right end of a quantal dose-response curve are referred to as___.

A. resistant
B. allergic
C. hyper-susceptible
D. reverse tolerant

49. The probit unit is used in a ___.

A. graded dose-response curve
B. quantal dose-response curve
C. both
D. neither

50. A sigmoid dose-response curve has the shape of ___.

A. inverted U
B. a straight line
C. an upright U
D. none of the above

51. A quantal dose-response curve ___.

   A. represents the response of one individual
   B. represents the response of a population
   C. cannot be used to calculate an LD50
   D. none of the above

CHAPTER 1 ANSWERS

1. A	28. D
2. C	29. A
3. C	30. B
4. D	31. C
5. D	32. A
6. C	33. A
7. A	34. B
8. A	35. A
9. B	36. B
10. A	37. B
11. B	38. C
12. D	39. C
13. C	40. C
14. D	41. B
15. A	42. D
16. B	43. B
17. C	44. D
18. B	45. D
19. D	46. A
20. C	47. C
21. C	48. A
22. D	49. B
23. C	50. D
24. B	51. B
25. B	
26. B	
27. B	

2

Absorption, Distribution, Excretion

52. All the following are necessary for a systemic toxic effect from a chemical except ___.

    A. absorption into the blood of the organism
    B. uptake into a target tissue
    C. biotransformation in the liver
    D. distribution from the site of absorption

53. All the following have natural barriers to toxicant penetration except ___.

    A. skeletal muscle
    B. brain
    C. placenta
    D. testes

54. The rate of penetration of a toxicant by passive diffusion into cells is related to ___.

    A. lipid solubility
    B. concentration gradient
    C. both
    D. neither

55. Which of the following is true regarding passive diffusion?

    A. It requires ATP.
    B. Chemicals can move against a concentration gradient.
    C. both
    D. neither

56. Which of the following is true regarding active transport?

    A. It requires energy.
    B. It is the most common way chemicals enter cells.
    C. both
    D. neither

57. The principal sight of absorption for gases in the respiratory tract is ___.

    A. trachea
    B. bronchus
    C. bronchioles
    D. alveolus

58. The rate of absorption of a gas in the lung is proportional to____.

    A. the solubility of gas in the blood
    B. the ionic radius of gas molecule
    C. both
    D. neither

59. The time to equilibrium between a gas in the alveolus and the dissolved gas in the blood is directly proportional to____.

    A. solubility of gas in the blood
    B. dielectric constant of gas molecule
    C. number of antibonding molecular orbitals on gas molecule
    D. none of the above

60. The passage of a toxicant into the brain is mostly related to its ____.

    A. water solubility
    B. lipid solubility
    C. melting point
    D. boiling point

61. A property of the blood – brain barrier cells that impairs the penetration of toxicants is ____.

    A. tight junctions with minimal pores
    B. waxy cell walls similar to plants
    C. both
    D. neither

62. An example of a chemical that exerts its toxic effect topically on the skin or gastrointestinal system is ___.

    A. a strong acid
    B. a strong base
    C. a strong oxidizer
    D. all the above

63. The passage of toxicants through the stratum corneum is by ___.

    A. active transport
    B. passive diffusion
    C. facilitated diffusion
    D. none of the above

64. The study of the time course of a toxicant in the body is called ___.

    A. toxicokinetics
    B. toxicodynamics
    C. dose – response
    D. concentration – effect relationship

65. If a toxicant is displaced from a plasma protein binding site there will acutely be a/an ___.

    A. decreased toxic effect
    B. no change in toxicity
    C. increased toxic effect
    D. increased toxic effect on the blood only

66. DDT stored in fat tissue, and lead stored in bone ___.

    A. can serve as depots for the toxicant
    B. are not toxic to fat and bone respectively
    C. both
    D. neither

67. A difference between active transport and facilitated diffusion is ___.

    A. active transport can go against a concentration gradient, whereas facilitated diffusion cannot
    B. active transport requires a carrier, whereas facilitated diffusion does not
    C. facilitated diffusion can be inhibited by a poison, whereas active transport cannot
    D. none of the above

68. Which of the following statements is true?

    A. Absorption through hair follicles is a major route of absorption through the skin.
    B. Skin in different parts of the body varies in its ability to absorb chemicals.
    C. The top layer of the skin is called the dermis.
    D. The dermis blocks penetration of chemicals better than the stratum corneum.

69. A protein constituent of plasma that binds chemicals is ___.

    A. Cytochrome A3
    B. deoxyribonucleic acid
    C. albumin
    D. cholesterol

70. Which of the following is true regarding sub-lingual absorption?

    A. Marketed drugs are absorbed this way.
    B. There is a large "first pass effect" by enzymes in the tongue.
    C. both
    D. neither

71. In the gastrointestinal tract, weak bases will best be absorbed through the ___.

    A. stomach
    B. esophagus
    C. rectum
    D. none of the above

72. Which of the following statements is/are true?

    A. Chemicals are more likely to be absorbed in the un-ionized form.
    B. Absorption of chemicals is possible through the rectum.
    C. both
    D. neither

73. Cell membranes are composed of ___.

    A. phospholipids
    B. embedded proteins
    C. both
    D. neither

74. Toxicants can pass through cell membranes by ___.

    A. transport through carriers
    B. penetration through pores
    C. cell engulfing
    D. all the above

75. The largest cellular pores occur in ___.

    A. capillaries
    B. muscle cells
    C. bone cells
    D. adipose cells

76. If an intravenous infusion of radiolabeled albumin were given to a human, the radioactivity would be ___.

    A. distributed equally throughout all organs of body tissues
    B. concentrated in bone
    C. confined mostly to the blood
    D. ah hundred percent eliminated in the urine within six hours

77. The blood brain barrier of a fetus ___.

    A. provides the same protection as an adult blood brain barrier
    B. does not allow methylmercury to penetrate
    C. both
    D. neither

78. The removal of a chemical by metabolism in the gut or liver after oral ingestion is called ___.

    A. intestinal pumping
    B. first pass effect
    C. reverse transport
    D. none of the above

79. Which of the following statements is/are true?

    A. The longer a chemical is in contact with part of the gastroin-
       testinal tract, the greater the systemic absorption.
    B. Particles can be absorbed through the gastrointestinal tract.
    C. both
    D. neither

80. Cells can engulf particles by the process of ___.

    A. phagocytosis
    B. pinocytosis
    C. both
    D. neither

81. Which of the following is considered parenteral absorption?

    A. intravenous
    B. rectal
    C. both
    D. neither

82. Which of the following is considered enteral absorption?

    A. intramuscular
    B. subcutaneous
    C. sublingual
    D. transdermal

83. Important carrier (transporter) systems for chemicals are located in ___.

    A. liver
    B. kidney
    C. both
    D. neither

84. The theoretical volume in which the total dose of administered drug would be uniformly distributed in the same concentration as plasma is called ___.

    A. total body water
    B. volume of distribution
    C. total body volume
    D. chemical volume

85. Which of the following statements is/are true?

    A. The placental barrier to toxicants can be made up of multiple cell layers
    B. Fluoride, lead, and strontium can concentrate in bone
    C. both
    D. either

86. If a toxicant concentrates in a non-target organ site such as adipose tissue, ___.

    A. the process can be protective against target organ toxicity
    B. a sudden loss of body fat from starvation can lead to toxicity
    C. both
    D. neither

87. Binding of toxicants to blood or tissue proteins is primarily through ___.

    A. non-covalent bonding
    B. metallic bonding
    C. both
    D. neither

88. Which of the following statements is/ true?

    A. Plasma is the fluid component of blood
    B. Serum is plasma without the fibrin clot
    C. both
    D. neither

89. The principal route of excretion for most toxicants is ___.

    A. bile
    B. exhalation
    C. urine
    D. gastrointestinal track

90. Which of the following statements is/are true?

    A. Most small molecule toxicants are filtered at the glomerulus
    B. Most polar toxicants are greater than 99% reabsorbed through the tubules
    C. both
    D. neither

91. Which of the following statements is/are true?

    A. Highly polar compounds are more likely to be excreted via the bile
    B. Compounds with molecular weights greater than 300 are more likely to be excreted via the bile
    C. both
    D. neither

92. Which of the following statements is/are true?

    A. An infant can ingest a toxicant through excretion into mother's milk.
    B. The liver and kidney have the ability to bind large amounts of chemicals
    C. both
    D. neither

93. Which of the following statements is/are true?

    A. Chemicals that are gases at body temperature are excreted via the lungs.
    B. Volatile liquids can be significantly excreted via the lungs.
    C. both
    D. neither

94. Which of the following types of chemical bonds usually results in higher toxicity when binding to biochemical molecules?

    A. ionic
    B. hydrogen
    C. van der wales
    D. covalent

95. If a toxicant is absorbed intravenously, ___.

    A. it is first distributed to highly perfused tissues
    B. it bypasses the "first pass effect"
    C. both
    D neither

96. Based on its large surface area, most toxicant absorption after oral ingestion occurs in the ___.

A. stomach
B. small intestine
C. large intestine
D. mouth and esophagus

97. A weak acid is mostly unionized in the ___.

A. small intestine
B. large intestine
C. stomach
D. rectum

98. A weak base is mostly unionized in the ___.

A. small intestine
B. large intestine
C. stomach
D. rectum

99. Which of the following statements is true?

A. Toxicants can be excreted into the urine by active secretion.
B. A highly lipid soluble toxicant is very likely to remain in the urine after glomerular filtration.
C. both
D. neither

100. A minor route of toxicant excretion is ___.

A. sweat
B. saliva
C. both
D. neither

CHAPTER 2 ANSWERS

52. C	79. C
53. A	80. C
54. C	81. A
55. D	82. C
56. A	83. C
57. D	84. B
58. A	85. C
59. A	86. C
60. B	87. A
61. A	88. C
62. D	89. C
63. B	90. A
64. A	91. C
65. C	92. C
66. C	93. C
67. A	94. D
68. B	95. C
69. C	96. B
70. A	97. C
71. D	98. A
72. C	99. A
73. C	100. C
74. D	
75. A	
76. C	
77. D	
78. B	

3

Biotransformation

101. In which of the following organs is biotransformation the least important ___.

    A. liver
    B. kidney
    C. lung
    D. pancreas

102. Biotransformation of a toxicant means ___.

    A. the metabolite is always more toxic than the parent
    B. the metabolite is always non-toxic
    C. the parent has no toxicity
    D. none of the above

103. The process of biotransformation involves ___.

    A. non-covalently binding chemicals to each other to form dimers and tetramers
    B. the chemical change of a parent molecule into a metabolite
    C. both
    D. neither

104. In general, biotransformation makes chemicals more ___.

    A. water-soluble

    B. lipid soluble

    C. acidic

    D. basic

105. A another term for biotransformation is ___.

    A. enzyme induction

    B. metabolism

    C. electron transport

    D. nuclear transformation

106. Most of the time biotransformation reactions result in ___.

    A. a metabolite that is more toxic than the parent

    B. a very lipid soluble molecule

    C. a metabolite that is less toxic than the parent

    D. an inorganic molecule

107. In the cell, biotransformation enzymes are located primarily in the ___.

    A. golgi apparatus

    B. nucleus

    C. endoplasmic reticulum and cytosol

    D. liposome

108. A compound that does not undergo significant biotransformation will accumulate ___.

    A. in the body
    B. in the environment
    C. both
    D. neither

109. In a phase 1 biotransformation reaction ___.

    A. nitric oxide is always released
    B. the molecule is usually made more polar
    C. a sugar molecule is added to the parent
    D. all the above

110. All the following are enzymes involved in phase 1 biotransformation reactions except ___.

    A. cytochrome P450
    B. flavin monooxygenases
    C. hydrolases
    D. glucuronosyltransferase

111. The endoplasmic reticulum fraction of a homogenized cell contains mostly ___.

    A. deoxyribonucleic acid
    B. microsomes
    C. ribonucleic acid
    B. none of the above

112. Which of the following is required in a reaction mediated by cytochrome P450 ?

    A molecular oxygen
    B NADPH
    C both
    D neither

113. Which of the following is true regarding cytochrome P 450?

    A There are many variants present in human liver cells.
    B It is located in the endoplasmic reticulum.
    C both
    D neither

114. An example of an aliphatic hydroxylation reaction is ___.

    A hexane to hydroxy-hexane
    B benzene to phenol
    C both
    D neither

115. Which of the following statements is/are true?

    A. Cytochrome P450 is only present humans.
    B. Cytochrome P450 is only present in liver.
    C. both
    D. neither

116. Which of the following statements is/are true?

    A. Reduction reactions are not considered phase 1 reactions.
    B. Reduction reactions are common in intestinal bacteria
    C. both
    D. neither

117. Which of the following statements is/are true?

    A. Cytochrome P450 enzymes are involved in the metabolism of endogenous hormones.
    B. Heme iron is reduced from the +3 state to +2 state during a cytochrome P450 mediated reaction.
    C. both
    D. neither

118. Which of the following statements is/are true?

    A. Cytochrome P450 is the same cytochrome involved in energy production in the electron transport chain.
    B. Cytochrome P450 is not present in forms of life lower than mammals
    C. both
    D. neither

119. The primary enzyme involved in the biotransformation of ethyl alcohol is ___.

    A. cytochrome P450 3A4
    B. methyltransferase
    C. alcohol dehydrogenase
    D. monoamine oxidase

120. Which of the following is not a cytochrome P450 mediated reaction?

    A. epoxidation
    B. hydroxylation
    C. sulfonation
    D. N-dealkylation

121. If and inorganic ion such as Mg+2 is required for an enzyme to work, the ion is referred to as a ___.

    A. coenzyme
    B. substrate
    C. cofactor
    D. coordination factor

122. Which of the following functional groups can be added as a result of a phase 1 biotransformation reaction ___.

A. -OH
B. -SiO2
C. both
D. neither

123. All the following are examples of phase 2 biotransformation reactions except ___.

A. epoxidation
B. acetylation
C. glucuronidation
D. methylation

124. A functional group that must be present for a glucuronidation reaction to occur is ___.

A. -SH
B. -OH
C. -COOH
D. all the above

125. The most common type of phase 2 reaction is ___.

A. oxidation
B. N-dealkylation
C. glucuronidation
D. hydrolysis

126. In humans, the most prevalent isoform of cytochrome P450 is ___.

    A. 2E1

    B 3A4

    C 2D6

    D 1A1

127. Phase 2 reactions in general will make a molecule ___.

    A. less polar

    B. smaller

    C. more lipid soluble

    D. more polar

128. Some biotransformation reactions occur at lower rates in ___.

    A. the elderly

    B. neonates

    C. both

    D. neither

129. The process by which the activity of a biotransformation enzyme can be greatly increased after exposure to an exogenous substance is called ___.

    A. enzyme induction

    B. enzyme multiplication

    C. enzyme enhancement

    D. enzyme magnification

130. Which of the following statements is true regarding inhibition of biotransformation enzymes?

    A. It can occur through the use of certain prescription drugs.
    B. It can occur after consuming grapefruit juice.
    C. both
    D. neither

131. The primary evolutionary purpose of biotransformation enzymes in humans was to ___.

    A. prevent the accumulation of toxic substances in the body
    B. produce different molecules that might be beneficial to digestive processes
    C. both
    D. neither

132. Many toxic electrophiles (positively charged molecules) are detoxified in the body by ___.

    A. glutathione
    B. Diels-Alder reaction
    C. Grignard reactions
    D. none of the above

133. Enzyme induction ___.

    A. requires a time delay for maximal effect

    B. involves the synthesis of new protein

    C. both

    D. neither

134. A prescription drug that induces its own biotransformation to a non-active metabolite would___.

    A. require a decrease in dosage over time to obtain the same pharmacologic effect

    B. require an increase in dosage over time to obtain the same pharmacologic effect

    C. require no change in dosage to obtain the same pharmacologic effect

    D. would require a decrease in dosage at the beginning, and the same dosage over time to obtain the same pharmacologic effect

135. Which of the following statements is/are true?

    A. Enzyme inducers of cytochrome P450 must be substrates for the enzyme.

j   B. Enzyme inhibitors of cytochrome p450 must be substrates for the enzyme.

    C. both

    D. neither

136. The activity of cytochrome P450 biotransformation enzymes can vary because of ___.

A. genetics
B. disease
C. cigarette smoking
D. all the above

137. Which of the following statements is/are true?

A. Each toxicant is bio-transformed to only one metabolite.
B. Peptides are more likely to be bio-transformed by cyto-chrome P450 than small molecules.
C. both
D. neither

138. Genetic polymorphisms can affect the activity of ___.

A. phase 1 biotransformation enzymes
B. phase 2 biotransformation enzymes
C. both
D. neither

139. Changes in the activity of biotransformation enzymes due to genetic polymorphisms can lead to ---.

A. increased risk of cancer
B. increased pharmacologic effect of a prescription drug
C. both
D. neither

CHAPTER 3 ANSWERS

101. D	128. C
102. D	129. A
103. B	130. C
104. A	131. A
105. B	132. A
106. C	133. C
107. C	134. B
108. C	135. D
109. B	136. D
110. D	137. D
111. B	138. C
112. C	139. C
113. C	
114. A	
115. D	
116. B	
117. C	
118. D	
119. C	
120. C	
121. C	
122. A	
123. A	
124. D	
125. C	
126. B	
127. D	

4

Toxicokinetics

140. The half-life of a toxicant refers to ___.

    A. the time it takes a toxicant to be 50 % absorbed from the body
    B. the time it takes for a toxicant to be 50 % eliminated from the body
    C. the time it takes for a toxicant to be 50 % eliminated from the environment
    D. after complete absorption, the time it takes for the plasma level of a toxicant to decrease by 50 %

141. If toxicant A has a half-life of two hours, and toxicant B has a half-life of four hours, then ___.

    A. it will take longer for toxicant A to reach steady-state
    B. it will take longer for toxicant B to reach steady-state
    C. toxicant A and B will reach steady-state at the same time
    D. toxicant A will reach steady state in 4 hours

142. The liver clearance of a toxicant is dependent on ___.

    A. liver blood flow
    B. activity of biotransformation enzymes
    C. both
    D. neither

143. Which of the following statements is/are true?

    A. The volume of distribution of a highly lipid soluble toxicant will always be higher than that of a highly water-soluble toxicant.
    B. For a highly lipid soluble toxicant, the concentration in fat tissue will always be higher than the concentration in plasma.
    C. both
    D. neither

144. In first order elimination kinetics, the slope of a semi-log concentration-time plot at the elimination portion of the curve is___.

    A. the absorption rate constant
    B. the excretion rate constant
    C. the elimination rate constant
    D. the redistribution rate constant

145. Total body clearance of a toxicant ___.

    A. is the sum of the individual organ clearances
    B. has units of volume per time
    C. both
    D. neither

146. A two compartment toxicokinetic model takes into consideration ___.

    A. distribution
    B. elimination
    C. both
    D. neither

147. In first order kinetics, if the dose of a toxicant is doubled___.

    A. the volume of distribution is doubled
    B. the total clearance is doubled
    C. both
    D. neither

148. In a 100 kg male patient, a toxicant with a volume of distribution of 1200 mL per kilogram would have a total body volume of distribution of ___.

    A. 12 L
    B. 120 L
    C. 1200 L
    D. none of the above

149. In drug or toxicant overdose situations, there may be___.

    A. saturation of biotransformation enzymes
    B. changes in clearance and half-life
    C. both
    D. neither

150. In first order kinetics, ___.

    A. total clearance is independent of dose
    B. elimination half-life is independent of dose
    C. both
    D. neither

CHAPTER 4 ANSWERS

140. D
141. B
142. C
143. C
144. C
145. C
146. C
147. D
148. B
149. C
150. C

5

Mechanisms of Toxicity

151. The process by which biotransformation creates a more toxic molecule from the parent molecule is called ___.

    A. conversion
    B. metabolic activation
    C. toxicant delivery
    D. systemic metabolism

152. Reabsorption of a toxicant back into the systemic circulation may take place ___.

    A. after biliary excretion
    B. in the renal tubules
    C. both
    D. neither

153. Enzymes participating in the detoxication of free radicals include ___.

    A. superoxide dismutase
    B. glutathione peroxidase
    C. both
    D. neither

154. The multidrug resistant protein transporter system ___.

    A. uses ATP
    B. transports toxicants into cells
    C. both
    D. neither

155. Which of the following statements is/are true?

    A. Different toxicologic mechanisms can contribute to a given toxic response.
    B. Different toxicologic responses can result from the same toxicologic mechanism.
    C. both
    D. neither

156. Superoxide anion radical and hydroxyl radical are examples of ___.

    A. cytokines
    B. reactive oxygen species
    C. both
    D. neither

157. All the following are types of toxic responses except ___.

    A. inflammation
    B. cell death
    C. cytochrome P450 inhibition
    D. carcinogenesis

158. Which of the following is the body's natural antioxidant?

A. folic acid
B. glutathione
C. vitamin D
D. cholesterol

159. Oxidative stress can cause toxicity to ___.

A. DNA
B. lipid membranes
C. both
D. neither

160. Reactive oxygen species can be produced by ___.

A. phagocytosis
B. the citric acid cycle
C. both
D. neither

161. Metal ions that may generate reactive oxygen species include ___.

A. Na and K
B. Mg and Mo
C. Fe and Cu
D. Ca and Bi

162. A common toxic response involving Ca+2 is ___.

    A. an increase in intracellular Ca+2
    B. a decrease in intracellular Ca+2
    C. conversion of Ca+2 to Ca+1
    D. conversion of Ca+2 to Ca radical

163. Heat shock proteins ___.

    A. can be present in small amounts in normal cells
    B. are produced as a homeostatic response to toxic cellular damage
    C. both
    D. neither

164. All the following statements are true regarding heat shock proteins except ___.

    A. they only function at a body core temperature greater than 103 degrees F
    B. they are also called molecular chaperones
    C. they are involved in normal protein folding
    D. they can carry old proteins to the proteasome (recycling bin)

165. When a toxic response overwhelms an adaptive or reparative response, the result can be ___.

    A. cell death
    B. fibrosis
    C. both
    D. neither

166. The process of apoptosis ___.

    A. rids the body of abnormal cells without an inflammatory response
    B. is another term for necrotic cell death
    C. both
    D. neither

167. All the following are involved in necrotic cell death except ___.

    A. cellular swelling
    B. need for ATP
    C. inflammatory response
    D. cell membrane rupture

168. All the following could cause necrotic cell death except ___.

    A. increase in intracellular Ca+2
    B. ATP depletion
    C. oxidative stress
    D. induction of biotransformation enzymes

169. Suppression of apoptosis could lead to ___.

    A. cancer
    B. decreased cell mass in an organ
    C. both
    D. neither

170. The Fas receptor ___.

    A. is a death receptor on the cell surface
    B. is involved in the process of apoptosis
    C. both
    D. neither

171. p53 is a protein that ___.

    A. can cause abnormal cells to undergo apoptosis
    B. can stop cellular proliferation in mutated cells
    C. is also called a tumor suppressor gene
    D. all the above

172. A person with a mutated p53 ___.

    A. will have a decreased risk of cancer
    B. will have decreased risk of atherosclerosis
    C. both
    D. neither

173. All the following are potential sites for a toxicant-receptor interaction except ___.

    A. G-protein coupled receptors
    B. ligand-gated ion channels
    C. voltage-gated ion channels
    D. albumin receptor

174. Decreased availability of ATP can occur with toxicants that affect___.

    A. mitochondria
    B. Citric acid cycle
    C. both
    D. neither

175. Which of the following can cause cell death by apoptosis?

    A. death receptor stimulation
    B. mitochondrial damage
    C. oxidative stress
    D. all the above

176. The cytochrome that is released from mitochondria and initiates cell death is ___.

    A. cytochrome A3
    B. cytochrome P450
    C. cytochrome c
    D. cytochrome P448

177. A mechanism by which toxicants affect mitochondria is ___.

    A. increased ATP production
    B. increase in the permeability of the mitochondrial inner membrane
    C. both
    D. neither

178. Repair to DNA ___.

    A. rarely happens
    B. is done solely by messenger RNA
    C. both
    D. neither

179. Toxicants can affect the immune system by ___.

    A. decreasing its function
    B. stimulating it
    C. both
    D. neither

180. Chemicals affecting transcription ___.

    A. can bind to intracellular receptors
    B. can be endocrine disruptors
    C. both
    D. neither

181. An important mechanism for tissue repair following toxicant exposure is ___.

   A. proliferation of adjacent normal cells
   B. suppression of apoptosis
   C. both
   D. neither

182. Cyanide anion is toxic by ___.

   A. disrupting the cytoskeleton of cells
   B. interfering with mitochondrial respiration
   C. both
   D. neither

183. Which of the following inhibits the citric acid cycle?

   A. digoxin
   B. atropine
   C. ketamine
   D. fluoroacetate

184. Which of the following is an inhibitor of the N-methyl -D-aspartate receptor?

   A. ketamine
   B. mercury
   C. morphine
   D. acetylcholine

185. Which of the following blocks the acetylcholine nicotinic receptor?

    A. tubocurarine
    B. benzodiazepines
    C. heroin
    D. naloxone

186. Which of the following is a frog toxin that acts opposite to tetrodotoxin?

    A. botulinum toxin
    B. batrachotoxin
    C. lophotoxin
    D. erabutoxin

187. Which of the following is a shellfish toxin that acts like tetrodotoxin?

    A. saxitoxin
    B. botulinum toxin
    C. cobrotoxin
    D. strychnine

188. Which of the following is a very potent toxin produced by anaerobic bacteria?

    A. tetanus toxin
    B. botulinum toxin
    C. both
    D. neither

189. All the following are inhibitors of mitochondrial electron transport except ___.

    A. serine
    B. rotenone
    C. MPP+
    D. hydrogen sulfide

190. Which of the following is a blocker of transmission at the neuromuscular junction?

    A. glucagon
    B. oxytocin
    C. both
    D. neither

191. Which of the following stimulates the release of catecholamines?

A. cocaine
B. methamphetamine
C. both
D. neither

192. Which of the following would speed up the heart rate?

A. atropine
B. epinephrine
C. both
D. neither

193. Which of the following would frequently cause seizures in overdose?

A. benzodiazepines
B. barbiturates
C. both
D. neither

CHAPTER 5 ANSWERS

151. B	178. D
152. C	179. C
153. C	180. C
154. A	181. A
155. C	182. B
156. B	183. D
157. C	184. A
158. B	185. A
159. C	186. B
160. A	187. A
161. C	188. C
162. A	189. A
163. C	190. D
164. A	191. C
165. C	192. C
166. A	193. D
167. B	
168. D	
169. A	
170. C	
171. D	
172. D	
173. D	
174. C	
175. D	
176. C	
177. B	

6

Testing Methods

194. All the following are true of acute toxicity testing except ___.

   A. It usually involves a single oral dose
   B. It cannot be done on airborne exposures
   C. It can involve intravenous or dermal exposures
   D. The LD50 is derived from the data

195. All the following are true regarding oral LD50 studies except ___.

   A. chemicals are usually administered in a vehicle
   B. sometimes chemicals can be added to the animal's food or water
   C. 5 to 15 grams/kg is usually a practical upper dosing limit
   D. control animals never receive vehicle

196. LD50 studies are usually performed in

   A. rat and mouse
   B. cat and dog
   C. primates
   D. rabbits

197. In rats that have decreased food consumption compared to controls, to establish that an adverse effect is due directly to the test chemical and not malnutrition, the toxicologist would usually___.

   A. switch the test animal
   B. feed the controls the same amount of food as the test ani-
      mals (pair-feeding)
   C. perform in vitro testing
   D. add vitamins to the food of the test animals

198. The regulation imposed by the FDA to insure the integrity of animal laboratory data is called___.

   A. Toxicology Practice Act (TPA)
   B. Laboratory Safety Act (LSA)
   C. Good Laboratory Practices (GLP)
   D. Good Clinical Practices (GCP)

199. All the following are true for chronic toxicity tests except___.

   A. they can last for the lifetime of the animal
   B. they are required in carcinogenesis studies
   C. they usually involve 2 to 3 test doses and a control
   D. one of the doses must be 75 % of the LD50

200. All the following are true for sub-chronic studies except ___.

    A. they are conducted primarily for toxicokinetics
    B. they can establish target organs
    C. they can establish a NOAEL
    D. they usually last 28 to 90 days

201. All the following are usually monitored at regular intervals in sub-chronic studies except ___.

    A. food consumption
    B. total body X-rays
    C. body weight
    D. behavior

202. Which of the following help to determine doses used in chronic toxicity studies?

    A. LD50
    B. slope of the acute dose-response curve
    C. results of a small 7-day dose-ranging study
    D. all the above

203. All the following are true in sub-chronic and chronic toxicity studies except ___.

    A. organs and tissues are examined histologically at the end
    B. blood is examined for hematology and chemistry
    C. half the animals are sacrificed on day 7
    D. urine is analyzed

204. A variable that could affect the results in animal toxicity studies is ___.

A. species
B. strain
C. age
D. all the above

205. Safety pharmacology studies are typically conducted to evaluate all the following target organs except ___.

A. heart
B. lung
C. bone
D. central nervous system

CHAPTER 6 ANSWERS

194. B
195. D
196. A
197. B
198. C
199. D
200. A
201. B
202. D
203. C
204. D
205. C

Carcinogenesis/Mutagenesis

206. Which of the following statements is/are true?

    A. A toxicant that causes cancer in laboratory animals will always cause cancer in humans
    B. Strong epidemiologic evidence of toxicant carcinogenesis in humans is more important than laboratory animal evidence
    C. both
    D. neither

207. A neoplasm can be___.

    A. a benign overgrowth of cells such as an adenoma
    B. a malignant overgrowth of cells such as a carcinoma
    C. both
    D. neither

208. Metastases are ___.

    A. cancer cells that have left the primary neoplastic site and spread to other organs
    B. cancer cells that are more sensitive to chemotherapy than the primary cells
    C. both
    D. neither

209. For a chemical to be considered mutagenic it must ___.

    A. damage or change genetic material
    B. damage or change phospholipids
    C. both
    D. neither

210. All the following are characteristics of genotoxic carcinogens except ___.

    A. mutagenicity
    B. reversibility
    C. dose-response relationship for tumor formation
    D. no threshold

211. All the following are characteristic of non-genotoxic carcino-gens except ___.

    A. no mutagenicity
    B. tissue specificity
    C. direct DNA damage
    D. reversibility

212. The initiation stage of carcinogenesis ___.

    A. always leads to a malignant tumor
    B. usually causes a mutation in DNA
    C. both
    D. neither

213. Initiated cells can ___.

    A. remain in a state of non-division
    B. undergo apoptosis
    C. divide and pass on the altered genetics
    D. all the above

214. Chemical agents initiate cancer commonly by ___.

    A. hydrogen bonding to DNA, forming chaperones
    B. covalently bonding to DNA, forming adducts
    C. both
    D. neither

215. Besides chemicals, initiation of carcinogenesis can be caused by ___.

    A. X-rays
    B. ultraviolet light
    C. viruses
    D. all the above

216. All the following are true regarding tumor promoters except ___.

    A. they are mutagenic
    B. they cause a clonal expansion of the initiated cell
    C. they may inhibit apoptosis
    D. they require continuous exposure to cause a pre-neoplastic growth

217. Which of the following statements is/are true regarding the progression stage of carcinogenesis?

    A. It is reversible.
    B. Benign pre-neoplastic cells are converted into cancer.
    C. both
    D. neither

218. Angiogenesis is ___.

    A. the formation of new structural protein around cancer
    B. the destruction of blood vessels supplying normal cells around cancer
    C. both
    D. neither

219. All the following are Hanahan and Weinberg properties of cancer except ___.

    A. sustained cell proliferation
    B. evading immume destruction
    C. inhibiting angiogenesis
    D. resisting apoptosis

220. A chemical that must be bio-transformed in the body to form a carcinogen is called a ___.

    A. ultimate carcinogen
    B. pro-carcinogen
    C. P450 carcinogen
    D. partial carcinogen

221. A chemical that can perform all three stages of carcinogenesis alone in called___.

    A. ultimate carcinogen
    B. proximate carcinogen
    C. complete carcinogen
    D. complex carcinogen

222. Most cancers ___.

    A. are formed from a single cell
    B. only need one mutation to be complete
    C. both
    D. neither

223. The reason for the increased incidence of human cancer with increasing age is ___.

    A. increase in immune system activity with age
    B. increased probability of multiple critical mutations with age
    C. both
    D. neither

224. Besides point mutations on DNA, chemicals that damage DNA can lead to ___.

    A. chromosome aberrations
    B. aneuploidy
    C. both
    D. neither

225. All the following are tumor promoters and not initiators except ___.

A. hormones
B. immunosuppressive drugs
C. high fat diet
D. histamine

226. Many genotoxic carcinogens are ___.

A. electrophilic
B. nucleophilic
C. both
D. neither

227. A type of normal gene that when mutated, can be converted to a gene that promotes cancer is called a/an ___.

A. oncogene
B. codon
C. growth factor
D. proto-oncogene

228. For a cancer to develop in an adult ___.

A. more than one gene must be mutated
B. the process usually requires a time span of over 20 years
C. both
D. neither

229. Tumor suppressor genes ___.

    A. inhibit cellular proliferation
    B. inhibit apoptosis
    C. both
    D. neither

230. All the following are tumor suppressor genes except ___.

    A. BRCA-1
    B. BRCA-2
    C. UDPGA
    D. P53

231. Tumors will most likely occur in mouse skin if ___.

    A. a promotor is used alone
    B. an initiator is applied after the promotor
    C. an initiator is applied alone
    D. a promotor is applied after an initiator

232. Which of the following factors is causal to the highest number of cancers?

    A. infections
    B. diet
    C. pollution
    D. medicines

233. Natural processes that oppose the development of cancer include ___.

    A. stopping the cell cycle so repair can take place

    B. apoptosis

    C. both

    D. neither

234. Which of the following statements is/are true?

    A. The incidence of human cancer plateaus at age 60.

    B. Several mechanisms for DNA repair exist.

    C. Most cancers form from a polyclonal group of cells.

    D. B and C

235. An important process that opposes the development of cancer is the process of ___.

    A. lipid repair

    B. DNA repair

    C both

    D. neither

236. A large percentage of human tumors contain mutations in the ____ oncogene.

    A. GDP

    B. NSAID

    C. RAS

    D. OATP

237. A theoretical chemoprevention drug against the formation of some types of cancer would be a/an ___.

    A. anti-apoptotic
    B. antioxidant
    C. both
    D. neither

238. The most popular short-term test for mutagenicity is the ___.

    A. Fick Test
    B. Retrovirus test
    C. Ames Test
    D. 2- year rodent carcinogenicity

239. In the IARC classification for human carcinogens, the agents with the most compelling evidence for causation are in Group ___.

    A. 1
    B. A
    C. 1A
    D. A1

240. A benign tumor must undergo ___.

    A. initiation
    B. promotion
    C. both
    D. neither

241. All the following are true of benzo{a}pyrene except ____.

    A. it is a procarcinogen
    B. it is metabolized in the body to an epoxide
    C. it is found in cigarette smoke
    D. it is an ultimate carcinogen

242. All the following are tests for mutagenicity except ____.

    A. Haber test
    B. Ames test
    C. mouse lymphoma assay
    D. Chinese hamster ovary test

243. The Ames test should be positive for a tumor ____.

    A. initiator
    B. promotor
    C. both
    D. neither

244. Human germ cells are ____.

    A. spermatozoa
    B. oocytes
    C. both
    D. neither

245. Inherited genetic damage is produced by mutations in ___.

    A. somatic cells
    B. germ cells
    C. both
    D. neither

246. A frame-shift mutation in DNA ___.

    A. will not alter the amino acid sequence of the translated protein
    B. occurs when the number of base pairs added or deleted is not a multiple of three
    C. both
    D. neither

247. Which of the following statements is/are true?

    A. The presence of micronuclei can indicate chromosomal damage.
    B. Chromosomal aneuploidy can involve an increase or decrease in the number of chromosomes.
    C. both
    D. neither

248. A chemical can be mutagenic by ___.

    A. altering DNA
    B. causing chromosomal aneuploidy
    C. causing chromosomal aberrations
    D. all the above

249. Chromosomal abnormalities are associated with ___.

    A. human birth defects
    B. human cancer
    C. both
    D. neither

250. All the following are complete carcinogens except ___.

    A. cigarette smoke
    B. estrogen
    C. asbestos
    D. radiation

CHAPTER 7 ANSWERS

206. B	233. C
207. C	234. B
208. A	235. B
209. A	236. C
210. B	237. B
211. C	238. C
212. B	239. A
213. D	240. C
214. B	241. D
215. D	242. A
216. A	243. A
217. B	244. C
218. D	245. B
219. C	246. B
220. B	247. C
221. C	248. D
222. A	249. C
223. B	250. B
224. C	
225. D	
226. A	
227. D	
228. C	
229. A	
230. C	
231. D	
232. B	

8

Developmental and Reproductive Toxicology

251. If a developing embryo is exposed to a toxicant during the zygote to blastula stage of development, the result could be ___.

   A. embryonic survival
   B. embryonic death
   C. both
   D. neither

252. If a fetus is exposed to a developmental toxicant, the likely result will be ___.

   A. cleft palate
   B. growth retardation and functional deficits
   C. heart valve abnormalities
   D. lung abnormalities

253. The period of organogenesis in humans is approximately ___.

   A. 10 to 20 days after conception
   B. 20 to 50 days after conception
   C. 50 to 70 days after conception
   D. 70 to 100 days after conception

254. Which of the following statements is/are true regarding teratogen exposure during the period of organogenesis?

A. Each organ system has a specific time interval during which it is vulnerable to teratogenicity.
B. A specific teratogen will only affect one specific organ system.
C. both
D. neither

255. An infectious agent that is teratogenic is ___.

A. roto virus
B. rhino virus
C. rubella virus
D. influenza virus

256. Female children of mothers exposed to diethylstilbestrol (DES) had an increased incidence of ___.

A. absent fingers
B. situs inversus
C. reproductive tract abnormalities
D. 3-chambered heart

257. An endocrine disruptor chemical could ___.

    A. mimic natural hormones
    B. antagonize natural hormones
    C. both
    D. neither

258. Exposure to an endocrine disruptor chemical in utero ___.

    A. will cause an increased sperm count in males
    B. will increase the risk of brain cancer in females
    C. both
    D. neither

259. Phthalates are endocrine disruptors found in ___.

    A. apples
    B. plastics
    C. pine wood
    D. soil

260. The fetal alcohol syndrome is associated with all the following except ___.

    A. neonatal cirrhosis
    B. intrauterine growth retardation
    C. craniofacial abnormalities
    D. impaired intellectual development

261. A vitamin that is teratogenic in higher than recommended doses is ___.

    A. vitamin A
    B. vitamin C
    C. vitamin E
    D. all the above

262. The progression of development in an embryo is largely dependent on numerous ___.

    A. cytokines
    B. transcription factors
    C. both
    D. neither

263. The progression of development in an embryo involves ___.

    A. apoptosis
    B. cell proliferation
    C. both
    D. neither

264. Male germ cell toxicity is opposed by ___.

    A. blood-testes barrier
    B. numerous ATP dependent efflux transporters
    C. both
    D. neither

265. All the following factors favor movement of a toxicant across the placenta except ___.

    A. high lipid solubility
    B. neutral charge
    C. substrate for an active transporter
    D. large molecular weight

266. A prescription drug that is a strong teratogen is ___.

    A. penicillin
    B. isotretinoin
    C. acetaminophen
    D. LSD

267. An example of a toxicant that could cause trans-placental carcinogenesis is ___.

    A. ethyl alcohol
    B. folic acid
    C. marijuana
    D. diethylstilbestrol (DES)

268. Which of the following statements is/are true regarding smoking and pregnancy?

    A. There is an increased risk of spontaneous abortions and lower birth weights.
    B. There is no increased risk of pregnancy problems from second hand smoke.
    C. both
    D. neither

269. Which of the following statements is/are true regarding cocaine use during pregnancy?

    A. It is strongly associated with retinoblastoma.
    B. Its presence can never be detected in a newborn.
    C. both
    D. neither

270. Which of the following statements is/ are true regarding radiation exposure and pregnancy?

    A. X-rays can be teratogenic
    B. exposure to ultraviolet-A light can be teratogenic
    C. both
    D. neither

271. All the following are used to evaluate reproductive toxicity in a male human except ___.

    A. voice quality
    B. blood testosterone levels
    C. sperm count
    D. sperm morphology

272. The in vivo animal developmental toxicology study that assesses fertility is ___.

    A. segment 1
    B. segment 2
    C. segment 3
    D. segment 4

273. The in vivo animal developmental toxicology study that assesses teratogenicity is ___.

    A. segment 1
    B. segment 2
    C. segment 3
    D. segment 4

274. Which of the following statements is/are true?

    A. Down's syndrome is caused by an abnormal number of chromosomes.
    B. Autism is caused by an abnormal number of chromosomes.
    C. both
    D. neither

275. Examples of in vitro developmental toxicology studies include using embryos of all the following
except ___.

    A. frogs
    B. slime molds
    C. zebrafish
    D. mice

276. The most famous teratogen that was a prescription drug initially approved in Europe and which caused limb abnormalities was ___.

    A. phenytoin
    B. valproic acid
    C. thalidomide
    D. losartan

277. Which of the following statements is/are true regarding development of the male external genitalia?

A. It is entirely dependent on the presence of testosterone and dihydrotestosterone during the 9th to 12th weeks of gestation.
B. Very rarely, XY chromosomal individuals will be insensitive to androgens, and female genitalia will result.
C. both
D. neither

278. Males exposed to endocrine disrupting chemicals that are estrogenic could have all the following when compared to non-exposed individuals except ___.

A. decreased sperm count
B. increased libido
C. lower serum testosterone levels
D. higher incidence of erectile dysfunction

279. A phytoestrogen ___.

A. is derived from a plant
B. is miroestrol.
C. can cause fertility problems in some animals
D. all the above

280. Endocrine disrupting chemicals that have recently been found to affect aquatic systems include ___.

   A. volcanic ash
   B. effluents from pulp and paper mills
   C. effluents from cattle concentrated animal feeding operations
   D. B and C

281. A dietary supplement that can prevent neurologic abnormalities and in the developing embryo is___.

   A. fish oil
   B. folic acid
   C. vitamin D
   D. vitamin B6

282. Laboratory animal male reproductive toxicity has been demonstrated by exposure to ___.

   A. pesticides
   B. zinc
   C. phthalates
   D. A and C

283. Human female reproductive toxicity has been demonstrated by exposure to ___.

    A. acetaminophen
    B. fluoride in toothpaste
    C. grapefruit juice
    D. none of the above

284. Which of the following statements is/are true?

    A. An embryo with many major malformations has a greatly increased risk of miscarriage.
    B. Approximately 3 percent of newborns will have major malformations.
    C. both
    D. neither

285. Endpoints for assessing the endocrine disrupting potential of a chemical in the rat include all the following except ___.

    A. electrocardiograms
    B. time of onset of puberty in females
    C. testes weight
    D. ovary weight

286. Proposed mechanisms for teratogenesis include all the following except ___.

A. DNA damage
B. increase in NADPH
C. formation of reactive oxygen species
D. hormonal interference

CHAPTER 8 ANSWERS

251. C	278. B
252. B	279. D
253. B	280. D
254. A	281. B
255. C	282. D
256. C	283. D
257. C	284. C
258. D	285. A
259. B	286. B
260. A	
261. A	
262. B	
263. C	
264. C	
265. D	
266. B	
267. D	
268. A	
269. D	
270. A	
271. A	
272. A	
273. B	
274. A	
275. B	
276. C	
277. C	

9

Immune System Toxicology

287. Which of the following statements is/are true?

    A. Immunodeficiency can lead to the development of cancer.
    B. Immunodeficiency can be congenital or acquired
    C. both
    D. neither

288. All the following are components of the innate immune system except ___.

    A. polymorphonuclear cells
    B. T cells
    C. macrophages
    D. complement

289. Innate immunity ___.

    A. does not need prior exposure to an infectious agent to help protect the organism
    B. does not have fever as a component.
    C. both
    D. neither

290. Toll-like receptors ___.

A. are on the surface of some cells involved in innate immunity ___.
B. recognize general characteristics of molecules present on microorganisms
C. both
D. neither

291. Mechanisms to prevent microbes from entering the human body include all the following except ___.

A. first pass metabolism
B. coughing
C. stomach pH
D. cilia in respiratory tract

292. Neutrophils can ___.

A. engulf invading microbes
B. release reactive oxygen species that help kill invaders
C. both
D. neither

293. All the following are true regarding thimerosal except ___.

A. it causes skin cancer in children
B. it contains mercury
C. it is a preservative
D it has been used for many years in vaccines

294. Macrophages ___.

    A. move from bone marrow to blood stream to tissues
    B. are called Kupffer cells in the brain
    C. both
    D. neither

295. All the following are true regarding the complement system except ___.

    A. it involves proteins found in blood
    B. it helps destroy bacterial cell membranes
    C. it participates in the inflammatory response
    D. it can induce phase 1 biotransformation enzymes

296. Antibodies are produced by ___.

    A. T cells
    B. basophils
    C. plasma cells
    D. monocytes

297. For antibodies to be produced, ___.

    A. a basophil must engulf an antigen
    B. a B cell must be presented with an antigen by a helper T cell
    C. both
    D. neither

298. The antibody found in secretions is ___.

A. IgM
B. IgG
C. IgA
D. IgD

299. The first antibody to appear following exposure to most antigens is ___.

A. IgM
B. IgG
C. IgA
D. IgD

300. The immune system can help defend an organism from ___.

A. viruses
B. cancer
C. both
D. neither

301. Histamine from mast cells in released in ___.

A. a type I allergic reaction
B. a type II allergic reaction
C. a type III allergic reaction
D. a type IV allergic reaction

302. T cells are primarily involved in a ___.

    A. type I allergic reaction
    B. type II allergic reaction
    C. type III allergic reaction
    D. type IV allergic reaction

303. Blood cells are attacked in a ___.

    A. type I allergic reaction
    B. type II allergic reaction
    C. type III allergic reaction
    D. type IV allergic reaction

304. Immune complexes are deposited in tissues in a ___.

    A. type I allergic reaction
    B. type II allergic reaction
    C. type III allergic reaction
    D. type IV allergic reaction

305. An anaphylactic reaction to a bee sting is a ___.

    A. type I allergic reaction
    B. contact dermatitis
    C. immune complex reaction
    D. none of the above

306. A rash from poison ivy is a ___.

    A. immediate hypersensitivity reaction
    B. T cell mediated reaction
    C. both
    D. neither

307. In penicillin allergy, a metabolite of penicillin acts as a ___.

    A. cytokine
    B. interleukin
    C. pyrogen
    D. hapten

308. Which of the following causes immunosuppression in humans?

    A. glucocorticoid hormones
    B. phenobarbital
    C. both
    D. neither

309. Which of the following causes immunosuppression in laboratory animals and possibly humans?

    A. PCBs
    B. TCDD
    C. both
    D. neither

310. Skin contact with metallic nickel is associated with a high incidence of

    A. acne
    B. malignant melanoma
    C. contact dermatitis
    D. psoriasis

311. Which of the following statements is/are true regarding immunosuppression?

    A. It is needed in cases of organ transplantation.
    B. It can be produced by chemotherapeutic anti-cancer agents
    C. both
    D. neither

312. Which of the following statements is/are true regarding immune-stimulation?

    A. It can be useful in the treatment of certain cancers.
    B. Some agents that do this are called adjuvants.
    C. It can be produced by ionizing radiation exposure.
    D. A and B.

313. Which of the following is/are a reliable indicator of immune system toxicity in laboratory animals?

    A. increased pituitary weight
    B. atrophy of the thymus
    C. anemia
    D. B and C

314. Which of the following methods is/are used to measure a humoral immunity response in laboratory animals?

    A. Measurement of plasma concentrations of antibodies.
    B. Quantifying the number of B cells in the spleen.
    C. Plasma macrophage count
    D. A and B.

315. Which of the following statements is/are true regarding auto-immunity?

    A. It is defined as the inability to recognize self from non-self.
    B. Hundreds of chemicals and drugs have been proven to cause human autoimmune disease.
    C. both
    D. neither

316. Which of the following statements is/are true?

A. Immunostimulation can lead to infection and cancer.
B. Immunosuppression can lead to allergy and autoimmune disease.
C. both
D. neither

CHAPTER 9 ANSWERS

287. C
288. B
289. A
290. C
291. A
292. C
293. A
294. A
295. D
296. C
297. B
298. C
299. A
300. C
301. A
302. D
303. B
304. C
305. A
306. B
307. D
308. A
309. C
310. C
311. C
312. D
313. B

314. D
315. A
316. D

10

Hematologic Toxicology

317. All the following are cells found in the blood except ___.

A. red cells
B. eosinophils
C. Langerhans cells
D. platelets

318. The disease associated with a decreased amount of hemoglobin in red cells is called ___.

A. polycythemia
B. anemia
C. red cell hyperplasia
D. red cell hypertrophy

319. Young red blood cells are called ___.

A. schistocytes
B. bands
C. mylocytes
D. reticulocytes

320. A common cause of anemia worldwide is ___.

A. iron deficiency
B. radiation
C. both
D. neither

321. Which of the following in deficiency is associated with anemia ___.

A. vitamin B12
B. folic acid
C. both
D. neither

322. Anemias can result from ___.

A. decreased red cell production
B. increased red cell destruction
C. both
D. neither

323. A chemical that is toxic to bone marrow can produce decreased blood levels of

A. red cells
B. white cells
C. platelets
D. all the above

324. The formation of methemoglobin ___.

   A. shifts the hemoglobin-oxygen dissociation curve to the right
   B. involves the oxidation of heme iron to ferric iron
   C. both
   D. neither

325. Methemoglobin can form by exposure to ___.

   A. therapeutic drugs
   B. environmental chemicals
   C. both
   D. neither

326. The normal life span of a mature red blood cell is ___.

   A. 30 days
   B. 120 days
   C. 200 days
   D. 300 days

327. Certain drugs can bind to surfaces on red cell membranes and cause ___.

   A. increased red cell survival
   B. immune hemolytic anemia
   C. both
   D. neither

328. Oxidative hemolysis of red blood cells can be caused by a deficiency of ___.

A. DNA ligase
B. glucose 6 phosphate dehydrogenase
C. both
D. neither

329 An increase in blood eosinophils can occur in all the following except ___.

A. toxic oil syndrome
B. a syndrome associated with contaminated tryptophan
C. allergic reactions
D. bone marrow depression

330. Decreased neutrophil cell counts (neutropenia) can be caused by ___.

A. immunologic mechanisms
B. non-immunologic mechanisms
C. both
D. neither

331. Which of the following statements is/are true regarding acute myelogenous leukemia?

    A. It can be caused secondarily from exposure to penicillin antibiotics.

    B. It can be caused secondarily from exposure to anti-cancer medications.

    C. both

    D. neither

332. Thrombocytopenia can be caused by ___.

    A. decreased production of platelets

    B. increased destruction of platelets

    C. both

    D. neither

333. Drugs like aspirin reduce clotting by ___.

    A. decreasing the number of platelets

    B. decreasing the ability of the platelet to form a clot

    C. both

    D. neither

334. Warfarin affects coagulation by ___.

    A. inhibiting platelet function

    B. affecting fibrin clot formation

    C. both

    D. neither

335. Hematologic toxicity in laboratory animals can be assessed by ___.

A. pancreas biopsies
B. bone marrow biopsies
C. both
d. neither

CHAPTER 10 ANSWERS

317. C
318. B
319. D
320. A
321. C
322. C
323. D
324. B
325. C
326. B
327. B
328. B
329. D
330. C
331. B
332. C
333. B
334. B
335. B

Hepatic Toxicology

336. Nutrients from the gut enter the liver through the ___.

    A. portal artery
    B. hepatic artery
    C. portal vein
    D. hepatic vein

337. The phagocytic cell in the liver is called ___.

    A. hepatocyte
    B. stellate cell
    C. astrocyte
    D. Kupffer cell

338. The acinar zones in the liver differ in ___.

    A. the activity of cytochrome P450
    B. the concentration of oxygen
    C. distance from the blood supply
    D. all the above

339. The stellate cell ___.

A. stores fat
B. can secrete collagen scar tissue
C. both
D. neither

340. Bile ___.

A. contains bile acids, cholesterol, phospholipids, and other components
B. is necessary for adequate absorption of lipids from the small intestine
C. is made in hepatocytes
D. all the above

341. The liver is frequently a target organ for toxicity because ___.

A. it is one of the first organs exposed to oral toxicants.
B. it has a large amount of biotransformation enzymes
C. both
D. neither

342. The process of biliary excretion of a chemical and subsequent reabsorption into the blood is called ___.

A. first pass effect
B. biliary kinetics
C. intestinal cycling
D. enterohepatic cycling

343. Due to the incomplete ability of neonates to clear chemicals in the bile, they are in danger of developing increased levels of ___.

A. serotonin
B. lysine
C. bilirubin
D. vitamin C

344. The most common agent that causes fatty liver in humans is ___.

A. acetaminophen
B. ethanol
C. marijuana
D. cigarette smoke

345. The most common disease associated with fatty liver is ___.

A. Alzheimer's
B. emphysema
C. pneumonia
D. diabetes mellitus

346. A proposed mechanism for the development of fatty liver is ___.

A. increased production of triglycerides by the hepatocyte
B. impaired entry of triglycerides into the blood
C. both
D. neither

347. Which of the following statements is/are true regarding liver necrosis?

    A. It usually results from an acute insult.
    B. It almost always requires the victim to undergo liver trans-
       plantation for survival.
    C. It mostly involves the apoptosis of hepatocytes.
    D. A and B

348. The liver toxicity of carbon tetrachloride is thought to be due
to ___.

    A. the parent molecule
    B. chlorine gas
    C. production of a free radical
    D. B and C

349. Liver cell necrosis involves ___.

    A. rupture of the cell membrane
    B. consumption of ATP
    C. both
    D. neither

350. Acetaminophen causes liver necrosis by ___.

    A. biotransformation into aspirin
    B. formation of cyanide anion
    C. both
    D. neither

351. Toxicants requiring bioactivation to a toxic metabolite by CYP P450 2E1 metabolism will produce the greatest damage in the part of the liver ___.

    A. with the highest concentration of collagen
    B. with the highest concentration of bile acids
    C. with the highest concentration of cytochrome P450 enzymes
    D. A and C

352. Cholestasis ___.

    A. is increased production of bile
    B. is cessation or slowing of bile flow
    C. results in an elevation of bilirubin in the blood
    D. B and C

353. Many of the chemicals causing cholestasis ___.

    A. are environmental endocrine disruptors
    B. are prescription drugs
    C. both
    D. neither

354. Cirrhosis ___.

    A. is a response to inadequate repair
    B. leads to collagen deposition all over the liver
    C. both
    D. neither

355. Which of the following statements is/are true regarding the medical consequences of cirrhosis?

    A. it can double the size of the liver leading to organ compression
    B. it can cause decreased blood flow to hepatocytes
    C. both
    D. neither

356. The leading cause of cirrhosis in humans is ___.

    A. acute ethanol overdose
    B. chronic ethanol abuse
    C. occupational exposure to solvents
    D. occupational exposure to pesticides

357. A toxin from blue-green algae that damages the cytoskeleton of hepatocytes is ___.

    A. tetrodotoxin
    B. microcystin
    C. thrombin
    D. formic acid

358. A general anesthetic that has been associated with immune-mediated liver disease is

    A. halothane
    B. propofol
    C. lidocaine
    D. nitrous oxide

359. A mold toxin that has been associated with hepatocellular cancer is ___.

A. actin
B. aflatoxin
C. viscotoxin
D. grayanotoxin

360. An intermediate in the production of plastics that is associated with the rare angiosarcoma of the liver is ___.

A. diethyl ether
B. toluene
C. propene
D. vinyl chloride

361. All the following will be elevated in the blood of an individual with significant liver disease except ___.

A. acid phosphatase
B. aminotransferases (AST and ALT)
C. bilirubin
D. lactic dehydrogenase

362. Which of the following statements is/are true regarding the response of the liver to injury?

A. It can involve proliferation of hepatocytes.
B. It can involve proliferation of stem or oval cells
C. both
D. neither

CHAPTER 11 ANSWERS

336. C
337. D
338. D
339. C
340. D
341. C
342. D
343. C
344. B
345. D
346. C
347. A
348. C
349. A
350. D
351. C
352. D
353. B
354. C
355. B
356. B
357. B
358. A
359. B
360. D
361. A
362. C

Renal Toxicology

363. All the following statements are true of the renal cortex except ___.

    A. it receives 90% of total renal blood flow
    B. is the outermost part of the kidney
    C. toxicants delivered by the blood will more likely affect this area than other parts of the kidney
    D. is the area that contains the loop of Henle and collecting ducts

364. Which of the following statements is/are true regarding the renal glomerulus?

    A. It has large pores which allow chemicals with molecular weights under 60,000 to pass through
    B. It is located in the renal medulla
    C. both
    D. neither

365. All the following substances pass easily through the glomerulus except ___.

A. water
B. albumin
C. glucose
D. amino acids

366. All the following substances are usually almost completely reabsorbed through the renal tubules except ___.

A. glucose
B. amino acids
C. Na+
D. urea

367. All the following statements are true regarding the kidney
except ___.

A. it re-absorbs 75% of filtered water
B. it receives 20 to 25% of total blood flow
C. it produces 500 mL to 2500 mL of urine on average daily
D. it plays a major role in regulating the body's acid-base
   balance

368. Which of the following is/are not secretory functions of the kidney?

    A. regulation of thyroid hormone
    B. production of erythropoietin
    C. both
    D. neither

369. Which of the following areas of the kidney is exposed to high concentrations of toxicants through the process of forming a concentrated urine?

    A. glomerulus
    B. papilla
    C. Bowman's capsule
    D. efferent arteriole

370. Concentrations of toxicants may be very high in proximal tubular cells of the kidney due to ___.

    A. tubular secretion
    B. tubular reabsorption
    C. both
    D. neither

371. Which of the following is/are unusual mechanisms of renal toxicity?

   A. Chemicals may concentrate in arterioles causing renal emboli
   B. Chemicals may precipitate out in the tubular lumen causing damage and obstruction
   C. both
   D. neither

372. Which of the following statements is true regarding the reason hthe kidney is a frequent target organ for toxicants?

   A. high blood flow
   B. presence of biotransformation enzymes
   C. both
   D. neither

373. Secretory transporters for organic anions and cations are found in the ___.

   A. collecting duct
   B. proximal tubule
   C. both
   D. neither

374. Heavy metals may cause renal dysfunction by ___.

   A. binding to sulfhydryl groups on proximal tubule proteins
   B. interacting with the immune system to cause glomerular damage
   C. both
   D. neither

375. Aminoglycoside antibiotics may cause renal dysfunction by ___.

   A. damage to the proximal tubules
   B. precipitating out as renal stones
   C. both
   D. neither

376. All the following are functions of the kidney except ___.

   A. production of glucocorticoids
   B. regulation of blood pressure
   C. excretion of waste molecules and toxicants
   D. production of renin

377. Symptoms and signs of renal dysfunction include all the following except ___.

   A. decreased urine output
   B. protein in urine
   C. red cells in urine
   D. urea in urine

378. Which of the following statements is/are true regarding toxi-cant effects on the glomerulus?

   A. Most glomerular toxicants will increase glomerular filtration rate.
   B. Toxicants that interfere with the anionic charges on the glomerulus will cause the urinary excretion of large molecu-lar weight proteins
   C. both
   D. neither

379. Which of the following statements is/are true regarding the reason the kidney is a frequent target organ for toxicity?

   A. A toxicant can be in a low concentration in blood, but in a toxic concentration in the kidney.
   B. The pH 1 of the kidney can make weak acids more toxic.
   C. both
   D. neither

380. All the following are nephrotoxic metals except ___.

   A. mercury
   B. magnesium
   C. lead
   D. cadmium

381. Compensatory responses to injury of renal tubular cells include ___.

    A. reparative mechanisms in damaged cells.
    B. proliferation of un-damaged cells
    C. both
    D. neither

382. Which of the following statements is/are true regarding a chemical that will be a useful indicator of glomerular filtration rate?

    A. It must not be secreted or reabsorbed, and must be completely removed from plasma by glomerular filtration.
    B. Inulin clearance is a good parameter for glomerular filtration rate.
    C. both
    D. neither

383. Antidiuretic hormone works on ___.

    A. the collecting duct to produce a concentrated urine.
    B on the glomerulus to allow large molecules to be filtered
    C. both
    D. neither

384. Toxicant exposure to renal cells may cause cell death by the process of ___.

A. apoptosis
B. necrosis
C. both
D. neither

385. Analgesic nephropathy is due to long term use of ___.

A. opiate analgesics
B. non-steroidal anti-inflammatory drugs in combination with acetaminophen-like drugs
C. both
D. neither

386. The findings of red cells and high molecular weight proteins in the urine of a toxicant exposed individual suggests ___.

A. a urinary tract infection
B. glomerular damage
C. both
D. neither

387. The finding of glucose in the urine of a non-diabetic individual who has been exposed to a toxicant suggests ___.

    A. glomerular damage
    B. tubular damage
    C. both
    D. neither

388. A treatment for end stage chronic renal failure that can restore function back to normal is ___.

    A. free radical scavengers
    B. glucocorticoids
    C. immunosuppressants
    D. There is no medical treatment. The patient must have dialysis or a transplant.

389. Which of the following is true regarding alpha 2u-globulin nephropathy?

    A. It can be caused by unleaded gasoline in male rats.
    B. Humans cannot develop it.
    C. both
    D. neither

390. The finding of the low molecular weight protein beta-2-micro-globin in the urine is suggestive of damage to ___.

A. ureter
B. glomerulus
C. bladder
D. proximal tubule

391. Patients or laboratory animals with advanced renal disease will have increased serum levels of ___.

A. creatinine
B. blood urea nitrogen (BUN)
C. both
D. neither

392. An unusual example of a chemical that is made renal toxic after conjugation with glutathione is ___.

A. lithium
B. methanol
C. hexachlorobutadiene
D. ethylene glycol

CHAPTER 12 ANSWERS

363. D	390. D
364. A	391. C
365. B	392. C
366. D	
367. A	
368. A	
369. B	
370. C	
371. B	
372. C	
373. B	
374. C	
375. A	
376. A	
377. D	
378. B	
379. A	
380. B	
381. C	
382. C	
383. A	
384. C	
385. B	
386. B	
387. B	
388. D	
389. C	

Endocrine Toxicology

393. Toxicants affecting the function of the adrenal cortex may disrupt the production of ___.

    A. epinephrine
    B. glucocorticoids
    C. both
    D. neither

394. A tumor of the adrenal medulla that produces increased catecholamines is ___.

    A. prolactinoma
    B. glioblastoma
    C. pheochromocytoma
    D. insulinoma

395. Chemicals that inhibit thyroperoxidase will cause decreased production of ___.

    A. T4
    B. T3
    C. both
    D. neither

396. Chemicals that destroy parathyroid chief cells may cause ___.

  A. low levels of calcium in blood
  B. high levels of phosphate in blood
  C. both
  D. neither

397. Which of the following statements is true?

  A. Peptide hormones can bind to cell surface receptors to generate a response.
  B. Non-peptide hormones generally must enter cells to generate a response.
  C. both
  D. neither

398. All the following hormones have nuclear receptors except ___.

  A. estrogens
  B. androgens
  C. glucocorticoids
  D. insulin

399. Which of the following statements is/ are true regarding hormone-nuclear receptor interactions?

A. The receptor complex exits the cytosol and binds to cell surface receptors to elicit a pharmacologic response.
B. The receptor can enter the nucleus and affect transcription.
C. The receptor complex binds to DNA.
D. B and C

400. Which of the following are estrogen agonist endocrine disruptors?

A. 4-Nonylphenol
B. Kepone (chlordecone)
C. both
D. neither

401. Which of the following is consistent with exposure to an estrogen agonist endocrine disruptor?

A. increased anogenital distance in males
B. gynecomastia in males
C. increased prostate weight in males
D. all the above

402. Polybrominated biphenyl (PBB) exposure in humans has been associated with ___.

    A. angiosarcoma of the liver
    B. hypothyroidism
    C. both
    D. neither

403. Which of the following would be expected to cause decreased prostate and seminal vesicle weight after chronic exposure to laboratory animals?

    A. testosterone
    B. vinclozolin (fungicide)
    C. aldosterone
    D. epinephrine

404. Possible signs of endocrine disruption in humans include all the following except ___.

    A. decreased sperm count
    B. increase in violent crime
    C. early onset of puberty in girls
    D. delayed onset of puberty in boys

CHAPTER 13 ANSWERS

393. B
394. C
395. C
396. C
397. C
398. D
399. D
400. C
401. B
402. B
403. B
404. B

Toxicology of the Eye

405. The first line of defense against a toxicant entering the eye is ___.

    A. eyelash
    B. tear film
    C. iris
    D. lens

406. Which of the following has the highest penetration through the cornea?

    A. metal cations
    B. inorganic anions
    C. lipid soluble chemicals
    D. A and B

407. The space between the lens and retina is filled with ___.

    A. vitreous humor
    B. aqueous humor
    C. synovial fluid
    D. cerebral spinal fluid

408. Which of the following is least damaging to the cornea?

A. 0.1 N sulfuric acid

B. acetone

C. 0.1N potassium hydroxide

D. 0.1 M sodium chloride

409. An environmental factor causing lacrimation is ___.

A. photochemical smog

B. carbon monoxide

C. both

D. neither

410. A loss of transparency in the lens is called a/an ___.

A. vacuole

B. blind spot

C. cataract

D. infarct

411. Chronic administration of which of the following is most likely to cause an opacity in the lens ___.

A. aspirin

B. acetaminophen

C. erythromycin

D. glucocorticoids

412. The retinal toxicity of methanol is thought to be due to ___.

   A. methanol
   B. formaldehyde
   C. formic acid
   D. oxalic acid

413. A solvent that is toxic to the retina is ___.

   A. boric acid
   B. carbon disulfide
   C. normal saline
   D. B and C

414. The test in rabbits used to evaluate ocular irritancy is ___.

   A. Fick test
   B. capillary test
   C. Draize test
   D. Litmus test

415. Ocular toxic metals include ___.

   A. lead
   B. methyl mercury
   C. both
   D. neither

416. A blockade of drainage of the aqueous humor in the anterior chamber can produce ___.

    A. retinal vein thrombosis
    B. corneal detachment
    C. glaucoma
    D. cataracts

417. Drugs that can cause an acute rise in intraocular pressure include ___.

    A. anticholinergic drugs
    B. beta-blocking drugs
    C. both
    D. neither

418. Phototoxicity, or the absorption of light in the UV or visible spectrum by chemicals to produce toxic reactive intermediates, can occur in the ___.

    A. lens
    B. cornea
    C. retina
    D. all the above

419. Which of the following statements is/are true?

A. Detergents do not irritate the cornea because they cannot penetrate due to their hydrophilic properties.
B. Toxicants can affect color vision perception.
C. both
D. neither

420. Which of the following statements is/are true?

A. Systemically absorbed toxicants can never reach the eye.
B. Chemicals topically applied to the eye can never reach the systemic circulation.
C. both
D. neither

421. Which of the following statements is/are true?

A. The eye is capable of cytochrome P450 mediated biotrans-formation.
B. Intraocular melanin may concentrate toxicants in the eye.
C. both
D. neither

422. Which of the following statements is/are true?

A. Some toxicants can cause a peripheral neuropathy without affecting the ocular system
B. Cytotoxic cancer chemotherapy drugs can cause ocular toxicity.
C. both
D. neither

423. Which of the following statements is/are true?

A. Prolonged elevated oxygen levels can cause retinal damage.
B. Morphine can affect pupil size.
C. both
D. neither

424. Which of the following statements is/are true?

A. The cornea has a dual blood supply.
B. Chemicals are better absorbed through the conjunctiva than the cornea.
C. both
D. neither

CHAPTER 14 ANSWERS

405. B
406. C
407. A
408. D
409. A
410. C
411. D
412. C
413. B
414. C
415. C
416. C
417. A
418. D
419. B
420. D
421. C
422. C
423. C
424. B

15

Toxicology of the Skin

425. The major barrier to the entry of toxicants into the body through the skin is ___.

    A. dermis

    B. basement membrane

    C. stratum corneum

    D. subcutaneous fat

426. Which of the following statements is/are true?

    A. The outermost layer of the skin is composed of dead cells.

    B. The epidermis is thicker than the dermis.

    C. both

    D. neither

427. Toxicants can more readily enter the body through the skin if ___.

    A. they are dissolved in dimethyl sulfoxide (DMSO)

    B. the skin has a tattoo

    C. the skin is abraded

    D. A and C

428. Which of the following statements is/are true?

A. Chemicals can more readily enter the body through the skin if they are present under a   plastic occlusive wrap.
B. High molecular weight hydrophobic chemicals can penetrate the skin better than hydrophobic chemicals of low molecular weight.
C. both
D. neither

429. Which of the following skin diseases can make entry of toxicants through the skin easier?

A. seborrheic keratosis
B. hyperkeratosis
C. psoriasis
D. lentigo spots

430. Which of the following statements is/are true?

A. The skin lacks P450 biotransformation enzymes.
B. Drugs can be delivered to the systemic circulation by topical patches applied to the skin.
C. both
D. neither

431. A non-immune related reaction of the skin to a chemical on the skin is called ___.

    A. allergic dermatitis
    B. irritant dermatitis
    C. hypersensitivity reaction
    D. urticaria

432. When a chemical produces immediate coagulative necrosis and major tissue damage, the process is classified as a ___.

    A. hypersensitivity reaction
    B. contact dermatitis
    C. chemical burn
    D. deep irritant

433. An immune-mediated reaction to chemical exposure of the skin is called ___.

    A. hyperemic dermatitis
    B. marginal irritant dermatitis
    C. B cell dermatitis
    D. allergic contact dermatitis

434. Which of the following statements is/are true?

 A. Allergic contact dermatitis requires multiple contacts with the offending chemical.
 B. The degree of response to a chemical causing irritant dermatitis is proportional to the dose.
 C. both
 D. neither

435. UV-B radiation ___.

 A. is responsible for most of sun tanning.
 B. reaches the earth at 1000 times the level of UV-A radiation.
 C. both
 D. neither

436. Ultraviolet radiation interacting with the skin can ___.

 A. increase the levels of vitamin D
 B. lower elevated bilirubin levels in newborns
 C. both
 D. neither

437. Which of the following are associated with skin exposure to ultraviolet radiation?

 A. freckles
 B. squamous cell carcinoma
 C. skin tags
 D. A and B

438. Skin cancers have occurred after contact with ___.

    A. soot
    B. latex
    C. both
    D. neither

439. Which of the following statements is/are true regarding phototoxic dermatitis?

    A. It requires multiple exposures.
    B. It is more common than photoallergy
    C. The responsible chemicals interact with UV light to produce reactive oxygen or other free radicals.
    D. B and C

440. Which of the following statements is/are true regarding photoallergic dermatitis?

    A. It requires an incubation period after the first exposure
    B. It requires much higher doses of chemicals than phototoxicity.
    C. both
    D. neither

441. Which of the following statements are true regarding urticaria?

A. It is a type IV hypersensitivity reaction.
B. It involves the release of histamine and other chemicals from mast cells.
C. both
D. neither

442. Which of the following statements is/are true regarding latex allergy?

A. It is a type I hypersensitivity reaction.
B. Latex may contain proteins that cross react with food proteins, which would cause an individual to be more likely to develop food allergies.
C. both
D. neither

443. A potentially fatal disease which causes a severe necrosis of the epidermis is ___.

A. psoriasis
B. vitiligo
C. toxic epidermal necrolysis
D. rosacea

444. Which of the following skin areas has the most resistance to toxicant absorption?

A. skin on back
B. soles of feet
C. skin on face
D. skin on legs

445. A form of acne resulting from occupational exposure to chlorinated aromatic hydrocarbons is ___.

A. chemical acne
B. hair follicle acne
C. chloracne
D. dermal acne

CHAPTER 15 ANSWERS

425. C
426. A
427. D
428. A
429. C
430. B
431. B
432. C
433. D
434. C
435. A
436. C
437. D
438. A
439. D
440. A
441. B
442. C
443. C
444. B
445. C

Neurotoxicology

446. Which of the following statements is/are true?

    A. The autonomic nervous system is part of the peripheral nervous system.
    B. The autonomic nervous innervates glands and organs.
    C. both
    D. neither

447. All the following statements are true regarding the neuron except ___.

    A. dendrites receive information
    B. they do not contain a nucleus
    C. they can have multiple dendrites
    D. axons transmit information

448. A phagocytic cell in the central nervous system is ___.

    A. Schwann
    B. microglia
    C. astrocyte
    D. oligodendroglia

449. Which of the following are myelin producing cells?

    A. Schwann
    B. oligodendroglia
    C. both
    D. neither

450. All the following are functions of astrocytes except ___.

    A. structural support
    B. participation in the blood-brain barrier
    C. synthesis of myelin
    D. providing nutrients to neurons

451. Which of the following statements is/are true?

    A. Transmission of information down an individual neuron is by neurotransmitters.
    B. Transmission of information between neurons is mainly by electrical contact between cells.
    C. both
    D. neither

452. All the following are neurotransmitters except ___.

    A. glutamate
    B. acetylcholine
    C. lactate
    D. GABA

453. The postganglionic neurotransmitter for the sympathetic nervous system is ___.

    A. glycine
    B. lysine
    C. norepinephrine
    D. glucagon

454. The neurotransmitter at the neuromuscular junction is ___.

    A. epinephrine
    B. acetylcholine
    C. creatine
    D. glutamate

455. Which of the following statements is/are true regarding the blood-brain barrier?

    A. The endothelial cells of capillaries form tight junctions that impede the entry of chemicals.
    B. Schwann cells surround capillary cells to enforce the barrier.
    C. both
    D. neither

456. All the following statements are true except ___.

A. the blood-brain barrier can be damaged by toxicants.
B. many toxicants enter the brain by carriers designed to transport endogenous molecules.
C. the blood-brain barrier is diminished or absent in parts of the brain that produce hormones.
D. the capillary endothelial cells of the blood-brain barrier have increased ability for pinocytosis.

457. All the following statements are true except ___.

A. the resting potential of nerves is maintained by the Na+/K+ ATPase pump
B. ninety percent of the energy requirements of the nervous system are due to axonal transport
C. P-glycoprotein transporters inhibit the entry of chemicals into the brain
D. anterograde axonal transport carries organelles from the cell body to the axon

458. Myelin ___.

A. helps increase the speed of a nerve impulse.
B. is present in newborns at adult levels
C. both
D. neither

459. Which of the following would best penetrate the blood-brain barrier?

    A. tetanus toxin
    B. staphylococcus aureus toxin
    C. botulinum toxin
    D. methylmercury

460. Toxicants that affect synaptic transmission can ___.

    A. cause under-stimulation leading to paralysis
    B. cause overstimulation leading to seizures
    C. both
    D. neither

461. All the following statements are true except ___.

    A. the resting membrane potential is approximately -70mV
    B. repolarization begins with opening of bicarbonate channels
    C. the sodium-potassium pump restores the resting state of the neuron
    D. the nerve impulse starts at the dendritic part of the neuron

462. Saltatory conduction involves ___.

    A. an overall decrease in nerve conduction velocity
    B. action potential generation only at the Nodes of Ranvier
    C. both
    D. neither

463. Which of the following statements is/are true?

    A. GABA is an excitatory neurotransmitter
    B. glutamate is an inhibitory neurotransmitter
    C. both
    D. neither

464. Which of the following statements is/are true regarding neuronopathy except ___.

    A. there is a good chance for regeneration
    B. it is defined as death of the entire neuron
    C. both
    D. neither

465. All the following statements are true regarding axonopathies except ___.

    A. there is regional injury with sparing of the cell body
    B. there is no potential for repair in the peripheral nervous system
    C. usually the distal portions are affected by toxicants first
    D. myelin will often be affected along with the axon

466. All the following are true of Wallerian degeneration except ___.

A. it is a model for neurotransmitter related toxicity
B. experimentally, it involves slicing a nerve fiber in half
C. it causes degeneration of the axon distal to the injury
D. it causes swelling of the proximal portion of the axon

467. A chemical whose toxicity resembles Wallerian degeneration is ___.

A. sulfuric acid
B. hexane
C. para-amino-benzoic acid
D. ribose

468. Which of the following statements is/are true regarding axonopathy?

A. It may involve sensory nerves.
B. It may involve motor nerves.
C. both
D. neither

469. Tetrodotoxin ___.

A. is produced by chlamydia
B. enhances the action potential
C. both
D. neither

470. Toxins affecting the electrical activity of the nerves ___.

    A. can naturally be produced in fish and frogs
    B. can be produced by microscopic organism that fish eat
    C. both
    D. neither

471. The sodium ion channel can be affected by ___.

    A. certain pesticides
    B. GABA agonists
    C. both
    D. neither

472. All the following would cause neurotransmitter related toxicity except ___.

    A. cocaine
    B. amphetamine
    C. nicotine
    D. lithium

473. Which of the following is a chemical that was neurotoxic to premature infants after skin absorption?

    A. ethanol
    B. betadine
    C. hexachlorophene
    D. aloe vera

474. Symptoms of a peripheral neuropathy include all the follow-ing except ___.

    A. numbness
    B. seizures
    C. tingling sensation
    D. weakness

475. The action of acetylcholine at the synapse is terminated by ___.

    A. epoxide hydrolase
    B. acetylcholinesterase
    C. both
    D. neither

476. The action of acetylcholine at the muscarinic receptor synapse is blocked by ___.

    A. atropine
    B. physostigmine
    C. both
    D. neither

477. Inhibition of acetylcholine release is caused by ___.

    A. tetrodotoxin
    B. saxitoxin
    C. batrachotoxin
    D. botulinum toxin

478. Tetanus toxin ___.

    A. blocks the release of GABA and glycine
    B. blocks the release of epinephrine
    C. results in spastic paralysis
    D. A and C

479. All the following are useful testing procedures for assessing neurotoxicity in humans except ___.

    A. nerve conduction studies
    B. amino acids in urine
    C. neuropsychological evaluations
    D. evoked potentials

480. An overdose of an acetylcholinesterase inhibitor would cause toxicity at___.

    A. the neuromuscular junction
    B. sympathetic ganglia
    C. parasympathetic ganglia
    D. all the above

481. Which of the following gases is/are neurotransmitters?

    A. nitric oxide
    B. carbon monoxide
    C. both
    D. neither

482. The action of norepinephrine at the synapse is terminated by ___.

A. reuptake back into the axon
B. metabolism by P450 enzymes in the synaptic space
C. both
D. neither

483. GABA ___.

A. is a non-peptide neurotransmitter
B. affects chloride ion channels
C. is metabolized by monoamine oxidase (MAO)
D. A and B

484. All the following are neuropeptides except ___.

A. dopamine
B. enkephalin
C. oxytocin
D. vasopressin

485. Glycine ___.

A. is the main excitatory neurotransmitter of the CNS
B. is blocked by strychnine
A. is metabolized by catecholamine-O-methyltransferase
D. A and C

486. The NMDA receptor ___.

    A. is excitatory
    B. binds glutamate
    C. both
    D. neither

487. MPTP ___.

    A. is a pesticide
    B. causes a peripheral neuropathy
    C. causes a Parkinson's disease-like syndrome
    D. A and B

488. The phrase "mad as a hatter" arose from occupational exposure to ___.

    A. lead
    B. radium
    C. mercury
    D. carbon tetrachloride

489. Which of the following toxicant-toxicity pairs is incorrect?

    A. aspirin-ringing in the ears
    B. acetaminophen-dementia
    C. aminoglycoside antibiotics-hearing loss
    D. acrylamide-distal axonopathy

490. Which of the following tests is least useful in assessing neuro-toxicity in adult laboratory animals?

A. feeding behavior
B. weighing the brain
C. exploratory behavior
D. measurement of startle reflex

491. Which of the following are brain imaging technology that are helpful is assessing the effects of toxicants on the human brain?

A. computerized tomography (CT scan)
B. positron emission tomography
C. traditional X-ray of brain
D A and B

492. A test to measure the effect of toxicants on ion currents in neurons is ___.

A. evoked potentials
B. radioactive ligand binding studies
C. voltage clamp
D. electroencephalogram

493. Which of the following statements is/are true?

    A. Exposure of the developing nervous system to toxicants can have different effects compared to exposure while an adult.
    B. Damage to neurons in the CNS is followed by vigorous hyperplasia of neighboring neurons.
    C. both
    D. neither

494. In which of the following diseases is causation 100% due to environmental chemicals?

    A. Alzheimer's dementia
    B. multiple sclerosis
    C. Huntington's chorea
    D. none of the above

495. Which of the following statements is/are true?

    A. The nerve gas sarin works by stimulating glutamate receptors.
    B. Curare is a stimulant at the neuromuscular junction.
    C. both
    D. neither

CHAPTER 16 ANSWERS

446. C	473. C
447. B	474. B
448. B	475. B
449. C	476. A
450. C	477. D
451. D	478. D
452. C	479. B
453. C	480. D
454. B	481. C
455. A	482. A
456. D	483. D
457. B	484. A
458. A	485. B
459. D	486. C
460. C	487. C
461. B	488. C
462. B	489. B
463. D	490. B
464. B	491. C
465. B	492. C
466. A	493. D
467. B	494. D
468. C	495. D
469. D	
470. C	
471. A	
472. D	

17

Cardiovascular Toxicology

496. The cardiac cells that produce contractility are called ___.

    A. Purkinje cells
    B. cardiac fibroblasts
    C. myocytes
    D. actin cells

497. Which of the following statements is/are true?

    A. Oxygenated blood is pumped to the tissues by the left ventricle.
    B. Normal cardiac electrical activity originates at the tip of the left ventricle.
    C. both
    D. neither

498. Approximately what percent of cardiac cells are myocytes?

    A. 25%
    B. 40 %
    C. 65%
    D. 90%

499. Which of the following cells are involved in cardiac electrical impulse conduction?

A. sinoatrial node cells
B. atrioventricular node cells
C. Purkinje cells
D. all the above

500. Under normal circumstances, cardiac conduction originates in ___.

A. sinoatrial node cells
B. atrioventricular node cells
C. Purkinje cells
D. actin cells

501. Which of the following statements is/are true?

A. Heart rate can be increased by stimulation of the parasympathetic nervous system.
B. Heart rate can be decreased by stimulation of beta receptors in the sympathetic nervous system.
C. both
D. neither

502. Which of the following statements is/are true?

A. During normal growth and development, the heart grows primarily by division of myocytes.
B. In response to injury, the heart compensates by hypertrophy of myocytes.
C. both
D. neither

503. Which of the following cells is/are capable of spontaneous depolarizations?

A. Purkinje fiber cells
B. fibroblasts
C. both
D. neither

504. Which of the following is/are required for contraction of cardiac muscle?

A. ATP
B. calcium
C. both
D. neither

505. All the following statements regarding arrhythmias are true except ___.

    A. They can be caused by drugs or toxicants that affect the autonomic nervous system.
    B. Atrial arrhythmias are more ominous than ventricular arrhythmias.
    C. They affect the ability of the heart to pump blood efficiency.
    D. Ventricular fibrillation is the most serious.

506. All the following are involved in the generation of the cardiac action potential except ___.

    A. rapid inward movement of Na+
    B. rapid inward movement of Mg+2
    C. outward movement of K+
    D. Na+/K+ ATPase to restore the resting membrane potential

507. Coordination of electrical and mechanical activity in the heart is made possible by ___.

    A. blood-myocyte barrier
    B. electronic cell to cell coupling
    C. both
    D. neither

508. Which of the following are necessary for excitation-contraction coupling?

    A. interaction between actin and myosin
    B. ATPase
    C. both
    D. neither

509. A backup energy reserve molecule in the heart is ___.

    A. histidine
    B. arginine
    C. phosphocreatine
    D. lactate

510. Which of the following statements is/are true?

    A. Under normal circumstances, fatty acid oxidation provides the majority of energy for the heart.
    B. Under pathological conditions, anaerobic glucose metabolism increases.
    C. both
    D. neither

511. Damage to cardiac myocytes causing decreased contractility, leads to a condition called ___.

    A. systolic hypertension
    B. valvular heart disease
    C. heart block
    D. cardiomyopathy

512. Toxicant induced myocyte death can be caused by the process(es) of ___.

    A. necrosis
    B. apoptosis
    C. both
    d. neither

513. Which of the following statements is/are true?

    A. A decrease in cardiac muscle contractility can lead to congestive heart failure.
    B. Cardiac myocytes are similar to hepatocytes in that they have a large capacity to proliferate after damage.
    C. both
    D. neither

514. Which of the following statements is/are true?

    A. Alcohol is a significant cause of cardiomyopathy in many areas.
    B. Cardiac fibroblasts proliferate more than myocytes following injury.
    C. both
    D. neither

515. Halogenated hydrocarbons ___.

    A. cause accelerated blockage of coronary arteries.
    B. sensitize the heart to the arrhythmogenic effects of catecholamines.
    C. both
    D. neither

516. A blockage of a major coronary artery with resultant tissue ischemia and damage is called ___.

    A. cerebrovascular accident
    B. myocarditis
    C. ventricular hypertrophy
    D. myocardial infarction

517. The change in size, shape, structure, and function of the heart after injury to the heart muscle is called ___.

A. physiologic adaptation
B. cellular rearrangement
C. myocardial homeostasis
D. myocardial remodeling

518. The part of the electrocardiogram that when increased, is a risk factor for drug/toxicant induced ventricular arrhythmias is ___.

A. PR interval
B. P wave height
C. P wave width
D. QT interval

519. Toxicants that inhibit acetylcholinesterase could cause ___.

A. slow heart rate
B. hypotension
C. both
D. neither

520. Physiologic and adaptive myocardial hypertrophy ___.

A. can occur in response to exercise
B. occurs after birth
C. both
D. neither

521. Repair of cardiac muscle must involve ___.

    A. angiogenesis
    B. destruction of Pukinje fibers
    C. both
    D. neither

522. Cardiac glycosides like digoxin ___.

    A. can inhibit ATPase and can be used therapeutically to increase the force of cardiac contraction
    B. can cause ventricular ectopic beats and ventricular arrhythmias in overdose
    C. both
    D. neither

523. The anticancer drug doxorubicin (Adriamycin) is cardiotoxic because it ___.

    A. kills myocytes and causes a cardiomyopathy
    B. causes increased clotting leading to coronary artery occlusion
    C. damages the aortic valve leading to heart failure
    D. all the above

524. All the following events take place following a myocardial infarction except ___.

A. depletion of ATP
B change from aerobic to anaerobic metabolism
C. depletion of phosphocreatine
D. apoptosis of myocytes completely lacking ATP

525. Reperfusion of ischemic areas of the myocardium ___.

A. is the treatment of choice for myocardial infarction
B. may generate reactive oxygen species which can cause further damage
C. both
D. neither

526. Which of the following metals is least cardiotoxic?

A. sodium cation
B. cobalt
C. lead
D. cadmium

527. A sensitive blood marker of myocardial injury post myocardial infarction is ___.

A. acid phosphatase
B. creatine kinase BB
C. creatine kinase MB
D. alkaline phosphatase

CHAPTER 17 ANSWERS

496. C
497. A
498. A
499. D
500. A
501. D
502. B
503. A
504. C
505. B
506. B
507. B
508. C
509. C
510. C
511. D
512. C
513. A
514. C
515. B
516. D
517. D
518. D
519. C
520. C
521. A
522. C

523. A
524. D
525. C
526. A
527. C

18

Respiratory Toxicology

528. All the following are functions of the nose and nasal cavity except ___.

    A. warm incoming air
    B. trap nanoparticles
    C. provide smell receptors
    D. add moisture to the incoming air

529. Which of the following statements is/are true?

    A. Inhaled toxicants can rapidly enter the brain by passage through the olfactory epithelium.
    B. The nose can filter particles from 0.1 to 5 μm in diameter.
    C. both
    D. neither.

530. The flap of tissue that protects the airways from food or drink during swallowing is ___.

    A. larynx
    B. pharynx
    C. trachea
    D. epiglottis

531. All the following statements are true regarding alveolar epithelial cells except____.

  A. Clara cells contain P450 biotransformation enzymes
  B. type II cells cannot reproduce
  C. type II cells manufacture surfactant
  D. type I cells have a large surface area.

532. Which of the following statements is/are true?

  A. Macrophages are present in the alveoli.
  B. Type II cells play an important role in the response to toxicant-induced epithelial injury.
  C. both
  D. neither

533. Particles are cleared from the tracheobronchial region by the ____.

  A. islets of Langerhans
  B. mucociliary escalator
  C. both
  D. neither

534. Gas exchange between air and blood is decreased in situations of ___.

A. pulmonary edema
B. pulmonary fibrosis
C. both
D. neither

535. All the following cell types participate in an inflammatory response within the lung except ___.

A. neutrophils
B. macrophages
C. lymphocytes
D. microglia

536. Which of the following statements is/are true?

A. 95% of the oxygen in the blood is dissolved in the fluid of the blood.
B. In the tissues, the partial pressure of carbon dioxide is lower than the partial pressure of oxygen
C. both
D. neither

537. Which of the following statements is/are true regarding macrophages in the lung?

    A. They can engulf particles which are eventually eliminated by swallowing.
    B. In the process of defense, they can release mediators which can cause damage.
    C. both
    D. neither

538. Which of the flowing statements is/are true?

    A. Toxicants can affect the respiratory tract after being orally or intravenously ingested.
    B. Only gases can damage the alveolus.
    C. both
    D. neither

539. Toxicant induced spasm of the smooth muscle of the bronchioles is commonly called ___.

    A. asthma
    B. restrictive lung disease
    C. bronchitis
    D. pulmonary edema

540. During the repair process in the adult lung in response to a toxicant, an exaggerated growth factor stimulation of fibroblasts can produce ___.

A. pulmonary fibrosis
B. cystic fibrosis
C. both
D. neither

541. During the repair process in the adult lung in response to a toxicant, an exaggerated proteinase response may produce ___.

A. adenocarcinoma of the lung
B. emphysema
C. both
D. neither

542. The main site of absorption of most low water soluble toxicant gases is through the ___.

A. nasopharynx
B. esophagus
C. bronchioles
D. alveoli

543. Reactive oxygen species causing lung damage can be produced by ___.

    A. inhalation of ozone
    B. products of the inflammatory response
    C. particles containing metal oxides (Fenton and Haber-Weiss reactions)
    D. all the above

544. All the following are involved in antioxidant defenses in the lung except ___.

    A. superoxide dismutase (SOD)
    B. cytochrome P450 3F2
    C. catalase
    D. glutathione

545. Nanoparticles are deposited mainly in ___.

    A. nose
    B. pharynx
    C. bronchus
    D. terminal bronchioles and alveoli

546. Nanoparticles 0.1μm in size are deposited in the respiratory tract mainly by ___.

A. impaction
B. sedimentation
C. disintegration
D. diffusion

547. Which of the following statements is/are true regarding highly water soluble toxic gases like hydrochloric acid?

A. They cause most damage to the nasopharynx and trachea.
B. They dissolve in the mucus lining of the upper respiratory tract.
C. both
D. neither

548. A asthma-like syndrome that occurs after a single high dose exposure to a pulmonary irritant is called ___.

A. bronchiectasis
B. reactive airways dysfunction syndrome (RADS)
C. acute airway syndrome (AAS)
D. airway hypersensitivity syndrome (AHS)

549. Which of the following statements is/are true regarding hyper-sensitivity pneumonitis?

A. In contrast to asthma, it is a disease of the terminal bronchi-oles and alveoli.
B. The end result is lung cancer.
C. It can be initiated by exposures to molds and animal proteins.
D. A and C

550. The principal cause of chronic obstructive pulmonary disease is ___.

A. air pollution
B. cigarette smoking
C. mold exposure
D. solvent exposure

551. Asbestos exposure is associated with ___.

A. fibrotic lung disease
B. mesothelioma
C. both
D. neither

552. The hallmark of asthma is ___.

A. fibrosis
B. edema
C. increased elastase activity
D. bronchoconstriction

553. Which of the following statements is/are true regarding nanoparticles?

A. They may be absorbed into the blood through the respiratory system, and carried to other organs.
B. Carbon nanotubes are examples.
C. They have a large surface area to volume ratio.
D All the above.

554. All the following are associated with an increased risk of lung cancer except___.

A. carbon monoxide
B. cigarette smoke
C. second hand cigarette smoke
D. radon

555. Which of the following is/are cancer therapeutic agent(s) that causes pulmonary fibrosis?

    A. dexamethasone
    B. bleomycin
    C. both
    D. neither

556. Which of the following statements is/are true?

    A. Chronic silica dust exposure primarily causes obstructive lung disease.
    B. Toluene diisocyanate exposure primarily causes restrictive lung disease.
    C. both
    D. neither

557. Which of the following is least likely to cause pulmonary fibrosis?

    A. ammonia
    B. coal dust
    C. talc dust
    D. aluminum dust

CHAPTER 18 ANSWERS

528. B
529. A
530. D
531. B
532. C
533. B
534. C
535. D
536. D
537. C
538. A
539. A
540. A
541. B
542. D
543. D
544. B
545. D
546. D
547. C
548. B
549. A
550. B
551. C
552. D
553. D
554. A

555. B
556. D
557. A

19

Toxicology of Metals

558. Metals are considered unique toxicants because ___.

    A. most have antidotes
    B. they persist in the environment because they are elements
    C. once in the human body, they can never be eliminated
    D. they can be metabolized in the liver to metalloids

559. Which of the following statements is/are true?

    A. Metals are only toxic in the metallic state, and not as salts.
    B. The valance state of a metal can significantly affect its toxicity.
    C. both
    D. neither

560. All the following are significant sources of metal exposure except ___.

    A. volcanic eruptions
    B. groundwater contamination
    C. prescription sleeping pills
    D. fish consumption

561. Metal chaperones ___.

A. are involved with the movement of metals within cells
B. help prevent metal toxicity within cells
C. deliver metals into metalloproteins
D. all the above

562. Metal transporters ___.

A. transport metals across cell membranes
B. are involved in human diseases.
C. both
D. neither

563. Metallothionein ___.

A. detoxifies radon
B. can reduce the toxicity of certain metals
C. both
D. neither

564. All the following metals are essential for human well-being in the right amounts except ___.

A. titanium
B. iron
C. zinc
D. calcium

565. The principal route of lead exposure for young children is ___.

A. drinking water
B. household dust from older homes
C. food
D. stained glass

566. The target organ for lead toxicity in young children is ___.

A. liver
B. spleen
C. skin
D. central nervous system

567. All the following are major toxic effects of lead in adults except ___.

A. peripheral neuropathy
B. increase in red cell mass
C. hypertension
D. renal disease

568. Lead inhibits the enzyme ___.

A. catalase
B. delta-aminolevulinic acid dehydrase
C. cytochrome P450 3A4
D. cytochrome P450 1A2

569. The major hematologic effect of lead toxicity is ___.

    A. increased white cells

    B. decreased clotting

    C. increased platelets

    D. anemia with small cells

570. The clinically proven safe blood level in young children that prevents IQ and behavioral deficits is___.

    A. < 80 µg/L

    B. < 50 µg/L

    C. < 15 µg/L

    D. none of the above

571. The principal source of non-occupational mercury exposure in humans is ___.

    A. air pollution

    B. seafood consumption

    C. soil

    D. drinking water

572. The most toxic CNS form of mercury is ___.

    A. elemental mercury liquid

    B. methylmercury

    C. mercuric cation

    D. mercurous cation

573. The major target organ for mercuric mercury is the ___.

   A. liver
   B. bone marrow
   C. small intestine
   D. kidney

574. Which of the following statements is/are true?

   A. An open jar of elemental mercury left in a lab room for years is completely harmless.
   B. Oral ingestion of elemental mercury leads to death within minutes.
   C. both
   D. neither

575. Which of the following is/are instances of widespread accidental mercury exposure?

   A. Fish contamination in Minamata Japan.
   B. Rice contamination in Iraq and China.
   C. both
   D. neither

576. Which of the following statements is/are true regarding arsenic?

A. Like mercury, it can occur in organic and inorganic forms.
B. Arsenic has been shown to be a strong carcinogen in multiple laboratory animal species.
C. both
D. neither

577. The major source of non-occupational exposure to arsenic is ___.

A. air pollution
B. soil
C. dental implants
D. food and drinking water

578. All the following are target organs for acute inorganic arsenic toxicity except ___.

A. iris of eye
B. liver
C. heart
D. peripheral nervous system after 1 to 2 weeks

579. All the following skin diseases are associated with arsenic except ___.

   A. malignant melanoma
   B. basal cell carcinoma
   C. squamous cell carcinoma
   D. hyperkeratosis

580. Which of the following statements is/are true regarding arsenic?

   A. Phosgene is a toxic gas form of arsenic.
   B. Organic methylation of inorganic arsenic occurs in humans and other organisms.
   C. Arsenic accumulates in fingernails after chronic exposure.
   D. B and C

581. Which of the following statements is/are true regarding cadmium?

   A. It has a long half-life in the human body of possibly 10 to 30 years.
   B. Organic cadmium can cross the blood brain barrier and cause brain cancer.
   C. both
   D. neither

582. Cadmium will induce the formation of ___.

A. ferritin
B. albumin
C. metallothionein
D. B and C

583. An accidental human cadmium exposure in Japan led to ___.

A. blindness
B. very weak bones
C. erythema multiforme
D. brain cancer

584. Inhalation of cadmium is associated with ___.

A. obstructive lung disease
B. lung cancer
C. both
D. neither

585. Cadmium disease of the kidney affects ___.

A. glomeruli
B. tubules
C. both
D. neither

586. Which of the following is the least likely toxic reaction to nickel?

A. diabetes mellitus
B contact dermatitis
C. nasal carcinoma
D. lung carcinoma

587. Cobalt exposure has been associated with ___.

A. anemia
B. cardiomyopathy
C. both
D. neither

588. Which of the following statements is/are true?

A. Trivalent chromium is an essential trace element.
B. Hexavalent chromium is a carcinogen.
C. both
D. neither

589. Non-occupational exposure to lithium occurs primarily through ___.

A. drinking water
B. prescription pharmaceuticals
C. soil
D. air pollution

590. Which of the following would be least likely after lithium overdose?

A. renal disease
B. neurologic symptoms
C. hepatic necrosis
D. thyroid dysfunction

591. Manganese toxicity can produce some of the symptoms of ___.

A. iron deficiency
B. Parkinson's disease
C. both
D. neither

592. Wilson's disease is due to ___.

A. hepatic cooper accumulation
B. renal selenium accumulation
C. pancreatic antimony accumulation
D. none of the above

593. Iron overload can be caused by ___.

A. a hereditary condition causing increased intestinal absorption
B. multiple blood transfusions
C. both
D. neither

594. Aluminum accumulation in dialysis patients has been associated with ___.

A. squamous cell carcinoma of the skin
B. increased bicarbonate
C. dementia
D. dental caries

595. Bismuth is ___.

A. used in over the counter stomach medications
B. a frequent cause of human toxicity
C. both
D. neither

596. Beryllium ___.

A. inhalation can cause granulomatous disease of the lung
B. can cause a number of skin lesions
C. both
D. neither

597. Medicinal gold salts used to treat rheumatoid arthritis have been associated with ___.

A. immune complex glomerular disease
B. peptic ulcer disease
C. both
D. neither

598. Which of the following statements is/are true regarding tin compounds?

    A. Triethyltin and trimethyl tin are neurotoxic

    B. Inorganic tin compounds frequently cause myocardial infarction

    C. both

    D. neither

599. Gastroenteritis, polyneuropathy and baldness are hallmarks of ___.

    A. titanium poisoning

    B. fluorine poisoning

    C. thallium poisoning

    D. germanium poisoning

600. Irreversible pigmentation of the skin and eyes is associated with the toxicity of ___.

    A. thallium

    B. magnesium

    C. silver

    D. mercury

CHAPTER 19 ANSWERS

558. B	585. C
559. B	586. A
560. C	587. B
561. D	588. C
562. C	589. B
563. B	590. C
564. A	591. B
565. B	592. A
566. D	593. C
567. B	594. C
568. B	595. A
569. D	596. C
570. D	597. A
571. B	598. A
572. B	599. C
573. D	600. C
574. D	
575. C	
576. A	
577. D	
578. A	
579. A	
580. D	
581. A	
582. C	
583. B	
584. C	

20

Toxicology of Pesticdes

601. The most significant public health issue with pesticides is ___.

    A. massive human exposure through transportation accidents
    B. contamination of foods with pesticide residues
    C. development of pesticide resistance
    D. inhalation of pesticide residues in gardens

602. Which of the following statements is/are true?

    A. It usually takes 5 to 7 years of testing before a pesticide can be marketed.
    B. The US Food and Drug Administration (FDA) regulates pesticide use.
    C. both
    D. neither

603. All the following are classified as pesticides except ___.

    A. weed killers
    B. wood preservatives
    C. stucco paint
    D. fumigants

604. The ideal pesticide has ___.

    A. selective toxicity
    B. no environmental persistence
    C. both
    D. neither

605. Which of the following statements is/are true?

    A. Suicide by intentional ingestion of pesticides is a major problem in underdeveloped countries.
    B. The most commonly used pesticide class in the United States is herbicide.
    C. both
    D. neither

606. The mechanism of action of organophosphorus insecticides is ___.

    A. inhibition of norepinephrine release
    B. stimulation of dopamine receptors
    C. blocking Na/K ATPase
    D. inhibition of acetylcholinesterase

607. Some organophosphorous insecticides can cause ___.

    A. angiosarcoma of the liver

    B. delayed pulmonary fibrosis

    C. delayed neurotoxicity

    D. A and C

608. The mechanism of action of DDT-like pesticides is ___.

    A. inhibition of acetylcholinesterase

    B. interfering with voltage-gated sodium channels in the nerves of insects

    C. stimulating glycine release in insect brains

    D. B and C

609. Which of the following statements is/are true regarding DDT?

    A. It has lower human acute toxicity when compared to organo-phosphorous insecticides

    B. It is not useful to control mosquitos

    C. both

    D. neither

610. A class of insecticide that inhibits acetylcholinesterase is ___.

    A. carbamate

    B. cyclodienes

    C. chlorinated cyclohexane

    D. rotenoid

611. A naturally occurring pesticide present in chrysanthemum plants is ___.

    A. nicotine
    B. picrotoxin
    C. lindane
    D. pyrethrin

612. Beneficial properties of pyrethroids include ___.

    A. low environmental persistence
    B. low mammalian toxicity
    C. both
    D. neither

613. The herbicide 2, 4, dichloro-phenoxyacetic acid (2, 4-D) ___.

    A. kills grass but not most weeds
    B. works as an auxin regulator
    C. both
    D. neither

614. The major target organ for paraquat toxicity is the ___.

    A. bone marrow
    B. lung
    C. skin
    D. pancreas

615. A postulated mechanism for paraquat toxicity is ___.

    A. free radical formation followed by fibrosis

    B. inhibition of Na/K ATPase

    C. release of glutamate

    D. inhibition of cytochrome P450 3A4

616. The target organ for chronic exposure to diquat is ___.

    A. bone marrow

    B. spleen

    C. eye

    D. skeletal muscle

617. Agent orange is a mixture of ___.

    A. paraquat and diquat

    B. 2, 4 D and atrazine

    C. 2, 4 D and 2, 4, 5 T

    D. diquat and 2, 4, 5 T

618. TCDD ___.

    A. is a contaminant of agent orange manufacture

    B. is involved in controversies regarding its role in causing human cancer and birth defects

    C. exposure occurred to large populations during the Vietnam war

    D. all the above

619. Major concerns with the herbicide atrazine is/are ___.

    A. possible endocrine disruption in humans
    B. eye toxicity
    C. groundwater contamination
    D. A and C

620. Coumarin rodenticides work by ___.

    A. inhibiting Na/K ATPase
    B. inhibiting the inward Na current in rodent nerves
    C. enhancing the clotting system
    D. inhibiting the clotting system

621. All the following are true regarding the herbicide glyphosate except___.

    A. a trade name is Roundup
    B. it is one of the most commonly used pesticides in the United States
    C. its mechanism is to inhibit an enzyme necessary for the synthesis of aromatic amino acids in plants
    D. it is the most toxic herbicide still in use in the United States

622. The mechanism of fluoroacetate toxicity is ___.

    A. similar to tetrodotoxin
    B. similar to strychnine
    C. to disrupt the Krebs Cycle
    D. none of the above

623. Methyl bromide ___.

    A. is classified as a fumigant
    B. is relatively non-toxic to humans
    C. both
    D. neither

624. All the following are true of fungicides except ___.

    A. they help prevent crop loss
    B. they are used to kill molds in homes
    C. they can contaminate drinking water
    D. they are all highly toxic to mammals acutely

625. The intermediate syndrome is associated with exposure to ___.

    A. organophosphorus insecticides
    B. methyl bromide
    C. glyphosate
    D. B and C

626. All the following are true of neonicotinoid insecticide except ___.

    A. they have low mammalian toxicity
    B. they are agonists at the nicotinic acetylcholine receptor
    C. the principal target organ for acute toxicity in humans is bone
    D. their use has increased from year to year

627. All the following are insect repellants except ___.

A. alachlor
B. DEET
C. citronella
D. eucalyptus oil

628. The nerve gas sarin has a mechanism of action and chemical structure similar to ___.

A. organochlorine insecticides
B. organophosphorus insecticides
C. avermectins
D. nicotine

629. An example of a biopesticide is ___.

A. staphylococcus aureus
B. clostridium perfringens
C. bacillus thuringiensis
D. pseudomonas aeruginosa

630. Which of the following pesticide-pesticide class is incorrect?

A. DDT-herbicide
B. Chlorpyrifos-insecticide
C. 2, 4-D-herbicide
D. copper sulfate-fungicide

CHAPTER 20 ANSWERS

601. B	628. B
602. A	629. C
603. C	630. A
604. C	
605. C	
606. D	
607. C	
608. B	
609. A	
610. A	
611. D	
612. C	
613. B	
614. B	
615. A	
616. C	
617. C	
618. D	
619. D	
620. D	
621. D	
622. C	
623. A	
624. D	
625. A	
626. C	
627. A	

21

Chemical and Solvent Toxicology

631. Solvent abuse ___.

    A. can have the potential for tolerance and physical dependence
    B. is a worldwide problem
    C. causes a "high" by binding to vasopressin receptors
    D. A and B

632. The effect of solvents on the brain is similar to ___.

    A. ethanol
    B. barbiturates
    C. atropine
    D. A and B

633. Environmental contamination of solvents can occur in ___.

    A. drinking water
    B. the atmosphere around petroleum plants
    C the atmosphere around hazardous wastes sites
    D. all the above

634. Solvents can enter the body through____.

A. the skin
B. inhalation
C. gastrointestinal adsorption
D. all the above

635. Major routes of solvent elimination from the body include the following ____.

A. sweat
B. exhalation
C. metabolism
D. B and C

636. Many solvents are metabolized by ____.

A. rhodanese
B. acetylcholinesterase
C. cytochrome P450 2E1
D. cytochrome P450 2D5

637. All the following are true regarding trichloroethylene (TCE) except ____.

A. it is strongly associated with the development of glioblas-toma in humans
B. it was used as a metal degreaser
C. it may be associated with renal cell carcinoma in humans
D. it has contaminated groundwater

638. All the following are true regarding tetrachloroethylene (PERC) except ___.

    A. it is used in dry-cleaning
    B. it has contaminated groundwater
    C. it causes kidney cancer in male rats but human data on kidney cancer is inconclusive
    D. it floats on water

639. All the following are true regarding carbon tetrachloride except ___.

    A. its use has been steadily increasing since the 1970s.
    B. it is hepatotoxic and renal toxic in humans
    C. its toxic metabolite is a radical
    D. it was used as a fire extinguisher

640. All the following are true regarding chloroform except ___.

    A. it was formally used as an anesthetic
    B. it is not hepatotoxic
    C. it is metabolized to phosgene
    D. it is present in chlorinated drinking water

641. All the following are true regarding benzene except ___.

    A. it is present in gasoline
    B. it is present in cigarette smoke
    C. it is highly hepatotoxic
    D. it can cause leukemia in humans

642. All the following are true regarding toluene except ___.

    A. it is classified as a strong human carcinogen
    B. it is frequently used by solvent abusers
    C. the primary target organ is the CNS
    D. it is present in paints, thinners, glues and gasoline

643. All the following are true regarding ethanol except ___.

    A. it is a human carcinogen
    B. it accelerates atherosclerosis
    C. it is a recreational drink
    D. it is metabolized to acetaldehyde and acetic acid

644. All the following are true regarding methanol except ___.

    A. another name is wood alcohol
    B. it is metabolized to formic acid
    C. it is toxic to the retina
    D. its poisoning does not have an antidote

645. All the following are true regarding ethylene glycol except ___.

    A. it is present in automobile antifreeze
    B. it is more volatile than diethyl ether
    C. it is metabolized to oxalic acid which can precipitate out in the kidney
    D. it frequently poisons household cats and dogs because of its taste

646. All the following are true regarding carbon disulfide except ___.

    A. it is associated with an axonopathy
    B. it may cause cardiovascular disease
    C. welders have very high exposures
    D. carbon dioxide is one of its end metabolites

647. The major effect of organic solvents in general on the heart is ___.

    A. accelerated atherosclerosis
    B. valvular heart disease
    C. hyperplasia
    D. arrhythmias

648. All the following are true regarding formaldehyde except ___.

    A. it is an odorless gas
    B. it is a strong respiratory irritant
    C. detectable levels are often found in new homes
    D. it is a potential human carcinogen

649. All the following are true regarding acrylonitrile except ___.

   A. it is not carcinogenic in humans or animals
   B. it may produce hydrogen cyanide while burning
   C. rubber workers and acrylic fiber producers can be occupa-
   tionally exposed
   D. the treatment of acute poisoning is similar to that for cya-
   nide poisoning

CHAPTER 21 ANSWERS

631. D
632. D
633. D
634. D
635. D
636. C
637. A
638. D
639. A
640. B
641. C
642. A
643. B
644. D
645. B
646. C
647. D
648. A
649. A

Food Toxicology

650. All the following statements are true regarding GRAS substances except ___.

    A. it stands for "generally recognized as safe"
    B. the list was originally composed in 1958
    C. some heavy metals are on the list
    D. based on new toxicological information, the safety of some ingredients has recently been challenged

651. All the following statements are true regarding direct food additives except ___.

    A. the classification includes pesticide residues
    B. they are added to increase shelf life
    C. they are added to change the texture
    D. they are added to change the flavor

652. All the following statements are true regarding sulfites except ___.

    A. they are food colors
    B. they can prevent browning of fruits
    C. they are presently only used on processed foods
    D. they are associated with allergic reactions

653. All the following statements are true regarding butylated hydroxyanisole (BHA) except ___.

    A. its use has recently been banned due to cancer concerns
    B. it is an antioxidant
    C. it helps to prevent fatty foods from turning rancid
    D. it is a food additive

654. All the following statements are true regarding nitrates and nitrites except ___.

    A. they add color to meat
    B. they can form nitrosamines
    C. they can protect against botulism
    D. they can act as artificial sweeteners

655. Cyclamates ___.

   A. are no longer used in the United States due to some animal carcinogenicity results
   B. are artificial sweeteners
   C. are antioxidants
   D. A and B

656. Aspartame ___.

   A. is an amino acid analog
   B. is banned in the United States
   C. both
   D. neither

657. Saccharin ___.

   A. causes bladder cancer in rats which is thought to be irrelevant to humans
   B. is banned in the United states
   C. both
   D. neither

658. Indirect food additives ___.

   A. can come from chemicals in packaging material
   B. can be present from drugs given to farm animals
   C. both
   D. neither

659. Bisphenol A ___.

A. is an endocrine disruptor
B. is a yellow food color
C. can leach out of heated baby bottles that contain it
D. A and C

660. Phthalates ___.

A. have androgenic effects
B. are released into food from packaging
C. have been banned due to carcinogenicity concerns
D. A and C

661. Food contaminates ___.

A. can be intentionally added to foods
B. can be GRAS
C. both
D. neither

662. All the following are considered food contaminants except ___.

A. heavy metals
B. monosodium glutamate
C. pesticide residues
D. mycotoxins

663. Aflatoxin ___.

A. contaminates nuts and grains
B. is a potent liver carcinogen
C. is produced by a mold
D. all the above

664. Botulism from Clostridia botulinum comes from ___.

A. improperly canned food
B. vegetables contaminated with cow manure
C. both
D. neither

665. Monosodium glutamate ___.

A. is associated with "Chinese restaurant syndrome"
B. causes a hypersensitivity reaction
C. both
D. neither

666. The Delaney clause ___.

A. was added in 2010
B. involves the international shipping of foods
C. involves the carcinogenicity of food additives
D. involves the preservation of foods

667. The FDA position on the safety of traditional foods (not additives or contaminants) is ___.

    A. they must be proven safe
    B. the consumer must take the responsibility for safety, the FDA presumes nothing
    C. foods are presumed to be safe
    D. none of the above

668. Dietary supplements ___.

    A. unlike foods, must have "a reasonable expectation of causing no harm"
    B. are treated like prescription drugs in the eyes of the FDA
    C. both
    D. neither

669. When food causes a change in the level of a drug in the blood or the action of a drug, the process is called ___.

    A. food adverse reaction
    B food-drug interaction
    C. food intolerance
    D. food idiosyncrasy

670. Food allergy ___.

A. is more common with peanuts than peas
B. can lead to anaphylaxis
C. both
D. neither

671. Lactose intolerance is an example of ___.

A. food allergy
B. food poisoning
C. food idiosyncratic reaction
D. food hypersensitivity

672. All the following statements are true regarding scombroid poisoning except ___.

A. it involves histamine
B. it is a true anaphylactic reaction involving the immune system
C. it involves fish
D. it is classified as an anaphylactoid reaction

673. All the following are considered significant heavy metal contaminants of food except ___.

A. mercury
B. tungsten
C. cadmium
D. lead

674. All the following are significant halogenated hydrocarbon food contaminants except ___.

    A. tetrafluoromethane
    B. polychlorinated biphenyls (PCBs)
    C. polybrominated biphenyls (PBBs)
    D. polybrominated biphenyl ethers (PBDEs)

675. All the following are true regarding ciguatera poisoning except ___.

    A. it can result from consuming fish
    B. the toxin comes from microalgae
    C. it involves a neurotoxin
    D. it is almost always fatal

676. All the following are true regarding Staph food poisoning except ___.

    A. it requires treatment with antibiotics to resolve.
    B. it is caused by a toxin
    C. it results from keeping foods at room temperature
    D. the foods are inoculated with Staphylococcus aureus by food handlers after cooking

677. All the following are sources of pathogenic E. coli except ___.

    A. lettuce
    B. hamburger
    C. cow's milk
    D. contact with farm animals

678. The majority of food-related toxicity is due to ___.

    A. food additives
    B. food contaminants
    C. microbial contamination
    D. food allergy

679. Spongiform encephalopathies in humans like kuru are thought to be caused by ___.

    A. mycoplasma
    B. prions
    C. rickettsia
    D. chlamydia

680. All the following are true regarding genetically modified foods except ___.

A. they may contain genes that give them an advantage to resist insect damage
B. they are banned in Europe do to safety concerns
C. they are created by genetic engineering
D. they undergo safety studies to lower the risk of human health issues

681. The most rigorous safety testing for a new food additive would occur for ___.

A. FDA concern level I
B. FDA concern level II
C. FDA concern level III
D. FDA structure category A

CHAPTER 22 ANSWERS

650. C
651. A
652. A
653. A
654. D
655. D
656. A
657. A
658. C
659. D
660. B
661. D
662. B
663. D
664. A
665. C
666. C
667. C
668. A
669. B
670. C
671. C
672. B
673. B
674. A
675. D
676. A

677. C
678. C
679. B
680. B
681. C

23

Ecotoxicology

682. Abiotic degradation of a toxicant involves ___.

    A. photolysis
    B. hydrolysis
    C. both
    D. neither

683. All the following are true regarding biotic degradation of a toxicant except ___.

    A. it is usually much slower than abiotic degradation
    B. it can involve bacteria and fungi
    C. it occurs through the action of enzymes present in microorganisms
    D. its end products can be carbon dioxide, water, and minerals

684 All the following are true regarding nondegradative elimination processes except ___.

A. volatile chemicals can be moved by winds
B. sorption of chemicals to solids in a body of water can remove some of the toxicant from the water
C. toxicants in sediments are more likely to enter living organisms than those dissolved in water
D. sulfur can bind metals in sediments

685. All the following are proven examples of toxicant effects on natural selection except ___.

A. cigarettes causing lung cancer in humans
B. microorganisms becoming resistant to antibiotics
C. insects developing pesticide resistance
D. moths becoming less conspicuous due to soot

686. The most abundant and/or important species in a community is called ___.

A. major species
B. dominant species
C. principal species
D. crucial species

687. The tern biodiversity involves ___.

    A. the type of species in a community
    B. the number of species in a community
    C. both
    D. neither

688. Toxicants can affect the biodiversity of a community by ___.

    A. decreasing predators
    B. decreasing prey
    C. eliminating a dominant species
    D. all the above

689. Which of the following is the correct representation of energy flow in a community?

    A. primary producers to secondary producers to secondary consumers
    B. secondary producers to primary producers to secondary consumers
    C. primary consumers to primary producers
    D. producers to primary consumers to secondary consumers

690. Detritivores ___.

    A. are primary producers
    B. consume organic waste
    C. both
    D. neither

691. If a toxicant adversely affects the producer trophic level ___.

   A. there will be an increase in biomass in primary consumers
   B. there will be an increase in carnivore population
   C. both
   D. neither

692. All the following are important cycles in ecosystems except ___.

   A. nitrogen cycle
   B. silicon cycle
   C. carbon cycle
   D. hydrologic cycle

693. The longest residence time for a toxicant usually occurs in ___.

   A. air
   B. fresh water
   C. salt water
   D. soil

694. An example of environmental biotransformation reaction leading to increased toxicity of a chemical is ___.

   A. conversion of nitrate to nitrogen gas
   B. methylation of metals
   C. both
   D. neither

695. All the following are significant examples of toxicant effects on oceans except ___.

    A. oil spills
    B. plastic debris
    C. death of puffer fish releasing tetrodotoxin
    D. offshore dumping of hazardous waste

696. All the following toxicologically affect fresh water systems except ___.

    A. chelation of Na+ anion
    B. runoff of pesticides
    C. runoff of fertilizer
    D. presence of prescription and non-prescription drugs

697. All the following may occur as a result of increased CO_2 levels in the atmosphere causing climate change except ___.

    A. rise in sea level
    B. raising of ocean pH
    C. increase in average worldwide temperatures
    D. changes in precipitation

698. Biomagnification involves ___.

    A. increased toxicant concentration in one organ compared to another

    B. increase in organism toxicant concentration with movement up a food web

    C. both

    D. neither

699. Measurement of acetylcholinesterase activity as an assessment of pesticide toxicity on an organism is called a/an___.

    A. surrogate

    B. toxicity screen

    C. biomarker

    D. isomer

700. All the following are true regarding nanoparticles except?

    A. They can be 90 percent removed by the mucociliary escalator.

    B. They can be present in diesel exhaust and fireplace soot.

    C. They probably can pass through cell membranes

    D. They can deposit in the alveoli.

701. All the following are major air pollutants except ___.

    A. oxides of carbon

    B. oxides of silicon

    C. oxides of sulfur

    D. oxides of nitrogen

702. All the following are true regarding carbon monoxide except ___.

    A. it binds strongly to hemoglobin
    B. the antidote for exposure is amyl nitrite
    C. it reaches high levels in tunnels
    D. it major toxicity is neurological impairment

703. Carbon dioxide ___.

    A. is a greenhouse gas
    B. is a simple asphyxiant
    C. both
    D. neither

704. All the following are true regarding the greenhouse effect except ___.

    A. it occurs on the moon
    B. it is postulated to be a cause of climate change
    C. it involves trapping energy from the sun
    D. it involves more than one atmospheric gas

705. All the following are true regarding acid rain except ___.

    A. it can be produced from sulfur oxides
    B. it can be produced from ozone
    C. it can be produced from nitrogen oxides
    D. it can dissolve limestone

706. Global sulfur emissions ___.

    A. occur primarily from burning natural gas
    B. have declined since 1990
    C. both
    D. neither

707. All the following are true regarding ozone except ___.

    A. it is a primary pollutant from burning fossil fuels
    B. it has a beneficial effect in the upper atmosphere
    C. it is a human respiratory irritant
    D. it can be toxic to plants in high concentrations

708. The Montreal Protocol ___.

    A. regulates the use of ozone depleting chemicals
    B. only involves the United States
    C. both
    D. neither

709. Chlorofluorocarbons ___.

    A. act as a chemical catalyst in the chemical conversion of ozone to oxygen in the atmosphere
    B. are strong respiratory irritants
    C. were used as refrigerants
    D. A and C

710. All the following are true of particulate air pollution less than 1 mm in diameter except___.

    A. they are products of combustion
    B. they contain caustic alkaline chemicals
    C. they are respiratory irritants
    D. they may contain carcinogens

711. All the following are true regarding indoor air pollution except ___.

    A. effects on health can be immediate or may be delayed for years
    B. sources can include cigarette smoke, flooring, cleaning products, and heating systems
    C. radon is not considered an indoor air pollutant
    D. the problem has increased due to the construction of energy efficient homes

712. All the following are technologies designed to reduce air pollution except ___.

    A. catalytic converters on automobiles
    B. fracking
    C. flue gas scrubbers to remove sulfur oxides
    D. electrostatic precipitation devices

713. All the following are true regarding oil spills except ___.

    A. microorganisms can play a major part in the cleanup
    B. dispersing and diluting the oil has been proven to be the best cleanup tactic
    C. the immediate effects are on birds and mammals
    D. some scientists believe that human attempts at cleanup may be more harmful than beneficial

714. All the following are considered hazardous waste except ___.

    A. certain electronic devices
    B. helium from balloons
    C. nickel-cadmium batteries
    D. paint removers

715. Legionnaires' disease is in the category of ___.

    A. outdoor air pollutant
    B. building related illness
    C. water pollutant
    D. hospital acquired illness

716. All the following are components of photochemical air pollution except ___.

    A. ozone
    B. carbon monoxide
    C. aldehydes
    D. peroxyacetyl nitrates

717. All the following are true of asbestos except ___.

    A. it causes a rare tumor called mesothelioma
    B. it causes increased lung cancer rates in smokers
    C. it can cause non-cancerous lung disease
    D. it causes ocular cancer

718. All the following are significant pollutants of fresh water except ___.

    A. heavy metals
    B. methane
    C. pesticides
    D. fertilizers

719. All the following are true regarding thermal pollution except ___.

    A. the major source is from the sun shining on a waterway
    B. it can come from water used to cool a power plant
    C. it lowers the amount of dissolved oxygen in the water
    D. it can increase the rates of cellular respiration in aquatic organisms

720. All the following are true regarding eutrophication except ___.

    A. it is a decrease in nutrients in a water body
    B. it is associated with algae blooms
    C. it is frequently associated with the discharge of phosphates
    D. it can alter oxygen levels

CHAPTER 23 ANSWERS

682. C
683. A
684. C
685. A
686. B
687. C
688. D
689. D
690. B
691. D
692. B
693. D
694. B
695. C
696. A
697. B
698. B
699. C
700. A
701. B
702. B
703. C
704. A
705. B
706. B
707. A
708. A

709. D
710. B
711. C
712. B
713. B
714. B
715. B
716. B
717. D
718. B
719. A
720. A

24

Toxic Plants and Animals

721. Plant toxicants containing heterocyclic nitrogen rings are generally called ___.

    A. terpenes
    B. steroids
    C. alkaloids
    D. glucosides

722. All the following are toxicologically similar except ___.

    A. caffeine
    B. atropine
    C. theophylline
    D. theobromine

723. The foxglove plant contains ___.

    A. cocaine
    B. opium
    C. cardiac glycosides
    D. caffeine

724. Urushiol ___.

    A. is the irritant chemical in poison ivy

    B. is a potent neurotoxin

    C. both

    D. neither

725. Ricin is produced by ___.

    A. oleander

    B. azalea

    C. castor bean plant

    D. aster

726. Amanita phalloides is a toxic ___.

    A. algae

    B. evergreen

    C. mushroom

    D. flower

727. Amanita phalloides toxin causes ___.

    A. diarrhea

    B. liver damage

    C. both

    D. neither

728. Bitter almond seeds contain ___.

    A. formic acid
    B. cyanide
    C. bone marrow toxins
    D. all the above

729. The belladonna alkaloids cause ___.

    A. slow heart rate
    B. pinpoint pupils
    C. both
    D. neither

730. Capsaicin is useful in treating ___.

    A. arrhythmias
    B. chronic pain
    C. both
    D. neither

731. A carcinogenic plant is ___.

    A. ragwort
    B. bay laurel
    C. squill
    D. bracken fern

732. Ergot alkaloids ____.

    A. were used to treat migraine headaches
    B. are produced by a rye fungus
    C. both
    D. neither

733. Which of the following is responsible for the highest number of deaths and serious injuries per year?

    A. spiders
    B. scorpions
    C. millipedes
    D. carpenter ants

734. The bite of a black widow spider ____.

    A. produces a 10 cm or more characteristic skin lesion
    B. injects a neurotoxin
    C. both
    D. neither

735. The bite of a brown recluse spider ____.

    A. is greater than 50 percent fatal
    B. contains toxins consisting of multiple enzymes
    C. both
    D. neither

736. All the following are caused by tick bites except ___.

    A. yellow fever
    B. Lyme disease
    C. Rocky Mountain spotted fever
    D. ehrlichiosis

737. Formic acid is present in high concentrations in the venom of ___.

    A. spiders
    B. scorpions
    C. centipedes
    D. ants

738. Which of the following are true regarding bee stings?

    A. the venom contains histamine and enzymes
    B. 100 or more stings can be fatal
    C. both
    D. neither

739. The toxins of cone snails ___.

    A. target ion channels
    B. are non-peptides
    C. both
    D. neither

740. Tetrodotoxin is found in ___.

    A. Gila monster
    B. blue ringed octopus
    C. both
    D. neither

741. Which of the following are true regarding amphibian toxins?

    A. poison dart frogs contain batrachotoxin
    B. Toads can secrete bufotenin, a hallucinogen
    C. both
    D. neither

742. A toxic aquarium fish is ___.

    A. wrasse
    B. anthias
    C. lionfish
    D. clownfish

743. Bites from pit vipers commonly produce ___.

    A. local tissue effects
    B. pain
    C. both
    D. neither

744. Bites from coral snakes commonly ___.

    A. cause neurotoxicity
    B. do not cause death in the United States
    C. both
    D. neither

745. Paralytic shellfish poisoning results from ___.

    A. shellfish consuming a dinoflagellate
    B. saxitoxin or brevetoxin
    C. both
    D. neither

746. All the following animals produce toxins except ___.

    A. Gila monster
    B. platypus
    C. American wolf
    D. man-o'-war jellyfish

747. Snake venoms may contain all the following except ___.

    A. biogenic amines
    B. inorganic cations
    C. cyanide ion
    D. enzymes

748. Acute toxicologic effects from snake venoms include all the following except ___.

    A. pro-coagulation
    B. bleeding
    C. neurotoxicity
    D. diabetes mellitus

749. Antivenoms ___.

    A. are all created from human volunteers
    B. carry a risk of anaphylaxis
    C. both
    D. neither

CHAPTER 24 ANSWERS

721. C
722. B
723. C
724. A
725. C
726. C
727. C
728. B
729. D
730. B
731. D
732. C
733. B
734. B
735. B
736. A
737. D
738. C
739. A
740. B
741. C
742. C
743. C
744. C
745. C
746. C
747. C

748. D
749. B

25

Toxicology of Prescription and Over-the-Counter Medication

750. One antidote for cyanide overdose ___.

   A. is amyl nitrite
   B. works by forming methemoglobin
   C. both
   D. neither

751. The antidote for acetaminophen overdose is ___.

   A. amyl nitrite
   B. calcium chloride
   C. N-acetylcysteine
   D. potassium chloride

752. First generation tricyclic antidepressants in overdose can cause fatal ___.

   A. arrhythmias
   B. coronary thrombosis
   C. cerebral thrombosis
   D. metabolic alkalosis

753. The feared complication of acetaminophen overdose is ___.

    A. cardiomyopathy
    B. bone marrow depression
    C. hepatic failure
    D. lung cancer

754. A fatal complication of acute opiate overdose is ___.

    A. coronary thrombosis
    B. carotid artery dissection
    C. respiratory arrest
    D. cerebral thrombosis

755. The antidote for opiate overdose is ___.

    A. sodium bicarbonate
    B. potassium chloride
    C. naloxone
    D. saline

756. Which of the following statements is/are true regarding over -the counter medications?

    A. some were prescription medications in the past
    B. most "brand name" cough and cold preparations contain the same ingredients.
    C. both
    D. neither

757. All the following are potential treatments for drug overdose except ___.

    A. hyperthermia
    B. hemodialysis
    C. activated charcoal
    D. mechanical ventilation

758. Alkalinization of urine will result in increased body clearance of ___.

    A. weak bases
    B. weak acids
    C. neutral compounds
    D. none of the above

759. High dose vitamin C ___.

    A. can cure influenza
    B. should be part of a normal diet in pregnancy
    C. both
    D. neither

760. High dose vitamin A ___.

    A. can cause hepatitis
    B. can result from eating polar bear liver
    C. both
    D. neither

761. Which of the following statements is/are true?

   A. vitamin supplementation is usually necessary even in people who eat balanced diets
   B. fat soluble have a greater potential for toxicity compared to water soluble vitamins
   C. both
   D. neither

762. Adverse effects of cholesterol lowering statin medication include ___.

   A. liver toxicity
   B. skeletal muscle toxicity
   C. both
   D. neither

763. Cyanide anion causes toxicity by ___.

   A. disrupting the cytoskeleton of cells
   B. interfering with mitochondrial respiration
   C. both
   D. neither

764. Use of broad spectrum antibiotics can lead to ___.

   A. antibiotic resistance
   B. pseudomembranous colitis
   C. both
   D. neither

765. An overdose of a beta-blocker will cause ___.

A. hypertension
B. tachycardia
C. both
D. neither

766. Adverse effects of aspirin include ___.

A. tinnitus (ringing in the ears)
B. gastrointestinal bleeding
C. both
D. neither

767. All the following are true regarding isotretinoin (Accutane) except ___.

A. it causes birth defects in pregnant females
B. an adverse effect is dry lips
C. it causes birth defects in the offspring of male users
D. it can treat cystic acne

768. Nonsteroidal anti-inflammatory drug use is associated with an increased risk of ___.

A. heart attack and stroke
B. rheumatoid arthritis
C. both
D. neither

769. Overuse of nasal decongestants can cause ___.

    A. hypertension
    B. psoriasis
    C. both
    D. neither

770. The antidote to radioactive iodine after a nuclear disaster is ___.

    A. protamine
    B. potassium iodide
    C. calcium chloride
    D. thiamine

771. Antidotes for cholinesterase insecticide poisoning include ___.

    A. atropine
    B. 2-PAM
    C. both
    D. neither

CHAPTER 25 ANSWERS

750. C
751. C
752. A
753. C
754. C
755. C
756. C
757. A
758. B
759. D
760. C
761. B
762. C
763. B
764. C
765. D
766. C
767. C
768. A
769. A
770. B
771. C

26

Alcohol and Drug Abuse Toxicology

772. The lowest blood level of alcohol that is illegal while driving in most states is ___.

 A. 0.08 %
 B. 0.1 %
 C. 001 %
 D. 0.04 %

773. Which of the following statements regarding alcohol is true?

 A. blood levels of alcohol are usually lower than serum levels
 B. blood and serum levels of alcohol are usually equal
 C. blood levels of alcohol are usually higher than serum levels
 D. blood levels of alcohol are usually higher than plasma levels

774. All the following are field sobriety tests except ___.

 A. walk and turn
 B. one leg standing
 C. horizontal gaze nystagmus
 D. proverb reasoning

775. All the following are considered standard drinks except ___.

A. 1.5 ounce of 80 proof liquor
B. 12 ounces of beer
C. 5 ounces of wine
D. 1 ounce of malt liquor

776. Approximately how many grams of alcohol are contained in a standard drink?

A. 10
B. 14
C. 20
D. 25

777. All the following statements are true regarding cocaine except ___.

A. the smoked form is called crack.
B. the antidote is atropine
C. it blocks the reuptake of dopamine
D. it can act as a local anesthetic

778. The pharmacological actions of cocaine most resemble ___.

A. ketamine
B. amphetamine
C. phencyclidine
D. LSD

779. Which of the following are true regarding cocaine?

    A. tolerance to its effects develops over time
    B. its withdrawal syndrome is more severe than any other abused drug
    C. both
    D. neither

780. Benzodiazepines act by interacting with the _____ receptor.

    A. opiate
    B. cholinergic
    C. GABA
    D. dopamine

781. All the following are uses for benzodiazepines except ___.

    A. treating anxiety
    B. treating low blood pressure
    C. treating seizures
    D. treating insomnia

782. All the following are true regarding benzodiazepines except ___.

    A. overdose with benzodiazepines alone is much less dangerous than overdose of alcohol and benzodiazepines
    B. tolerance to the effects of benzodiazepines can develop
    C. a withdrawal syndrome to benzodiazepines can occur
    D. there is no antidote available for an overdose

783. All the following are effects of amphetamine except ___.

    A. anorexia

    B. increased alertness

    C. decrease in blood pressure

    C. increase in heart rate

784. A drug pharmacologically similar to phencyclidine is ___.

    A. tetrahydrocannabinol

    B. ketamine

    C. fentanyl

    D. lorazepam

785. Phencyclidine acts primarily on the ___ receptor.

    A. NMDA

    B. cannabinoid

    C. cholinergic

    D. GABA

786. Some people who abuse phencyclidine have symptoms resembling ___.

    A. Parkinsons's disease

    B. multiple sclerosis

    C. schizophrenia

    D. diabetes

787. All the following act on the opioid receptor except ___.

    A. codeine
    B. fentanyl
    C. methamphetamine
    D. heroin

788. The antidote for opiate overdose ___.

    A. will produce withdrawal symptoms in addicts
    B. can be administered intramuscularly or subcutaneously in an emergency
    C. both
    D. neither

789. Withdrawal from opiates can be treated with all the following except ___.

    A. methadone
    B. methamphetamine
    C. buprenorphine
    D. clonidine

790. Endogenous molecules that bind to the opioid receptor are called ___.

    A. cytokines
    B. endorphins
    C. complements
    D. clotting factors

791. The active metabolite of heroin is ___.

A. morphine
B. fentanyl
C. meperidine
D. methadone

792. Heroin is a preferred opiate in addicts because ___.

A. it is safer than morphine
B. it enters the brain rapidly
C. both
D. neither

793. The drug with the dubious distinction of being called "date rape drug" is ___.

A. ketamine
B. chloral hydrate
C. phenobarbital
D. gamma-hydroxybutyrate

794. All the following are hallucinogens except ___.

A. LSD
B. propoxyphene
C. mescaline
D. psilocybin

795. Which of the following is considered to be a unique effect of MDMA?

    A. it is safe in overdose
    B. it makes you feel "empathy"
    C. it makes you see sounds
    D. it is present naturally in humans

796. Which of the following is the best definition of tolerance?

    A. the elimination of adverse effects and retention of beneficial effects
    B. the need for escalating drug doses to obtain the same initial effect
    C. the development of a severe physical withdrawal syndrome after discontinuation
    D. the psychological need to continue the drug

797. Which of the following statements is/are true regarding amphetamines?

    A. they can be synthetized from non-sedating over-the counter antihistamines
    B. users do not develop tolerance
    C. both
    D. neither

798. All the following are effects of amphetamines except ___.

A. psychosis
B. excitement
C. hyperthermia
D. pinpoint pupils

799. Delta-9-tetrahydrocannabinol (THC)

A. acts on specific receptors in the brain
B. cannot be absorbed orally
C. both
D. neither

800. All the following are typical effects of THC except ___.

A. nausea
B. blood-shot eyes
C. decreased intraocular pressure
D. bronchodilation

801. Which of the following is/are true regarding THC?

A. an overdose can cause psychosis
B. methamphetamine is an antidote for overdose
C. both
D. neither

802. Which of the following do many hallucinogens have in common?

    A. they are chemically glycosides
    B. they act on serotonin receptors
    C. both
    D. neither

CHAPTER 26 ANSWERS

772. A
773. A
774. D
775. D
776. B
777. B
778. B
779. A
780. C
781. B
782. D
783. C
784. B
785. A
786. C
787. C
788. C
789. B
790. B
791. A
792. B
793. D
794. B
795. B
796. B
797. D
798. D

799. A
800. A
801. A
802. B

27

Forensic and Analytical Toxicology

803. The process that causes the concentration of a chemical in a postmortem blood sample to be higher than the value at the time of death is called ___.

A. postmortem contamination
B. reverse entropy
C. reverse equilibrium
D. postmortem redistribution

804. Chemicals commonly used in criminal poisonings include all the following except ___.

A. arsenic
B. cyanide
C. strychnine
D. biotin

805. Which of the following have been used to measure postmortem concentrations of toxicants and drugs?

    A. insect larvae

    B. vitreous humor

    C. hair

    D all the above

806. Which of the following is/are true regarding the postmortem analysis of sample for chemicals?

    A. nonvolatile organics are most commonly measured

    B. volatile substances can't be measured

    C. both

    D. neither

807. The most accurate analysis of forensic samples is obtained from ___.

    A. thin -layer chromatography

    B. radio immunoassay

    C. acid titration

    D. GC-MS

808. A routine urine drug screen would detect the presence of all the following except ___.

   A. cocaine
   B. amphetamine
   C. THC
   D. arsenic

809. The burden of proof standard in a criminal poisoning is ___.

   A. preponderance of evidence
   B. beyond reasonable doubt
   C. reasonable medical certainty
   D. reasonable medical probability

810. Which of the following are true regarding urine drug screens?

   A. false positives can be reported
   B. time of ingestion can be accurately determined
   C. both
   D. neither

811. The analytical technique that involves placing samples at the bottom of a silica gel glass plate and allowing organic solvents to move up the plate by capillary action is called ___.

   A. thin-layer chromatography
   B. gas chromatography
   C. liquid chromatography
   D. mass spectrometry

812. The analytical technique that involves a liquid stationary phase on packed particles is called ___.

    A. thin-layer chromatography
    B. gas chromatography
    C. liquid chromatography
    D. mass spectrometry

813. The analytical technique that involves a stationary phase of solid particles and a liquid mobile phase is called ___.

    A. thin-layer chromatography
    B. gas chromatography
    C. liquid chromatography
    D. mass spectrometry

814. Which of the following analytical techniques involve the use of a specially prepared antibody?

    A. RIA
    B. EMIT
    C. both
    D. neither

815. Which of the following opiates would not be detected by a routine urine drug screen that detects the opiate ring structure ___.

A. heroin
B. morphine
C. methadone
D. codeine

816. All the following are clues that a recently collected urine specimen has been adulterated except ___.

A. yellow-orange color
B. specific gravity of 1.000
C. temperature of 76 degrees F
D. pH of 2.0

CHAPTER 27 ANSWERS

803. D
804. D
805. D
806. A
807. D
808. D
809. B
810. A
811. A
812. B
813. C
814. C
815. C
816. A

28

Radiation Toxicology

817. Radiation that carries enough energy to remove electrons from the outer orbitals of atoms is called ___.

  A. long wave radiation
  B. quantum radiation
  C. ionizing radiation
  D. photon radiation

818. Particles that carry enough energy to interact with biologic tissue include all the following except ___.

  A. graviton
  B. alpha particles
  C. beta particles
  D. neutrons

819. All the following are ionizing radiation except ___.

  A. X-rays
  B. gamma rays
  C. extreme short wave ultraviolet
  D. radio waves

820. Which of the following cell types is least likely to be affected by radiation?

    A. rapidly dividing cancer
    B. cardiac myocyte
    C. intestinal lining cell
    D. bone marrow

821. The energy from radiation can interact with DNA and cause ___.

    A. double strand breaks
    B. more efficient repair of DNA damage
    C. both
    D. neither

822. Linear energy transfer ___.

    A. is a measure of the energy transferred to biologic tissue per distance traversed
    B. depends of the energy of the radiation
    C. depends on the path length traveled
    D. all the above

823. Which of the following has the lowest linear energy transfer?

    A. X-ray
    B. alpha particle
    C. proton
    D. neutron

824. An instrument that can record the amount of radiation that an individual is exposed to is called ___.

   A. screening badge
   B. dosimeter
   C. lumen counter
   D. chromatograph plate

825. All the following are natural sources of radiation except ___.

   A. radon
   B. ozone
   C. potassium-40
   D. uranium-238

826. Atomic bomb survivors ___.

   A. had an increased risk for solid tumors
   B. had an increased risk for leukemia
   C. both
   D. neither

827. The unit of radiation exposure called the Sievert (Sv) takes into consideration ___.

   A. energy absorbed by biologic tissue
   B. a weighing factor to compare different forms of radiation
   C. both
   D. neither

828. Human information regarding radiation risk exposure can be obtained from all the following groups except ___.

   A. uranium miners
   B. patients with multiple X-rays for ankylosing spondylitis
   C. welders
   D. nuclear power workers

829. High radon levels in homes increases the risk for ___ cancer.

   A. colon
   B. lung
   C. both
   D. neither

CHAPTER 28 ANSWERS

817. C
818. A
819. D
820. B
821. A
822. D
823. A
824. B
825. B
826. C
827. C
828. C
829. B

Risk Assessment

830. The number of new cases of a disease in a fixed time period is called ___.

    A. disease proportion
    B. prevalence
    C. relative disease rate
    D. incidence

831. The number of cases of a disease per population number at a fixed time point is called ___.

    A. incidence
    B. disease per capita
    C. prevalence
    D. absolute disease rate

832. A model of a hypothetical straight-line relationship between sets of 2 variables is ___.

    A. parabolic fit
    B. simple linear regression
    C. correlation equation
    D. first derivative

833. A correlation coefficient of 0.9 would indicate ___.

    A. strong correlation
    B. weak correlation
    C. no correlation
    D. inverse correlation

834. Combining the results of 2 or more statistical studies to show that a difference exists between groups is called ___.

    A. analysis of variance
    B. meta-analysis
    C. group correlation
    D. statistical merging

835. All the following are statistical tests except ___.

    A. Student's t-test
    B. analysis of variance
    C. Chi Square-test
    D. Litmus test

836. The amount of chemical that is considered safe when ingested on a daily basis for a lifetime is called ___.

    A. daily safe dose (DSD)
    B. lifetime safe dose (LSD)
    C. acceptable daily intake (ADI)
    D. daily threshold dose (DTD)

837. Cohort studies ___.

A. are prospective
B. involve humans exposed and not exposed to a particular agent
C. both
D. neither

838. Case-controlled studies ___.

A. are retrospective
B. compare humans with a disease to non-diseased individuals
C. both
D. neither

839. The reference dose is the NOAEL ___.

A. divided by an uncertainty factor greater than 1
B. multiplied by a modifying factor greater than 1
C. both
D. neither

840. The air concentration of a chemical which is believed to be safe for a worker to be exposed to on a daily basis for a lifetime is called___.

A. toxic daily limit (TDL)
B. threshold limit value (TLV)
C. toxic ceiling limit (TCL)
D. threshold toxic limit (TTL)

841. The air concentration of a chemical which is believed to be safe for a worker to be exposed to for a 15-minute period is called ___.

    A. short term exposure limit (STEL)
    B. acute toxicity limit (ATL)
    C. toxic short-term limit (TSTL)
    D. acute toxic ceiling (ATC)

CHAPTER 29 ANSWERS

830. D
831. C
832. B
833. A
834. B
835. D
836. C
837. C
838. C
839. A
840. B
841. A

Essay/Short Answer Questions

GENERAL PRINCIPLES

842. *Explain the meaning of "the dose makes the poison".*

This statement was first made by Paracelsus, and has become the basic principle of modern toxicology. It means that any substance (even common substances that are essential for life like water and salt) can be toxic at high enough doses. It also means that common poisons like mercury and arsenic can be completely non-toxic if the dose or exposure is small enough. A recent addition to this adage is the principle that the rate at which a human being is exposed to toxic substance is also related to its poison potential. This concept is especially relevant for patients receiving intravenous drugs.

843. *Explain the difference between a graded and quantal dose-response curve.*

In a graded dose-response curve, dose is plotted on the X-axis, and the response of an individual is plotted on the Y-axis. In a quantal dose-response curve, an "all or none" response to a toxicant in a population is plotted on the Y-axis, and usually the logarithmic dose is plotted on the X-axis.

844. *Explain the difference between the NOEL and LOAEL.*

The NOEL, or no effect level, is the highest dose on a dose-response curve where there is no observable adverse effect. The LOAEL is the lowest dose on the dose-response curve where there is an observable adverse effect.

845. *Explain hormesis and give a clinically relevant example.*

Hormesis is a phenomenon in which low doses of a chemical have a beneficial effect up to a certain threshold, then increasing doses become toxic. Vitamin consumption at low doses can prevent deficiency diseases in certain individuals, but at high doses can be toxic.

ABSOPBTION, DISTRIBUTION, EXCRETION

846. *Explain why DDT persists in the environment and the human body?*

DDT has two properties that make it very likely to persist in the human body and the environment. It is very fat-soluble, and resistant to human biotransformation. The carbon – chlorine bond is very strong and resists metabolic degradation both in living organisms and in the outside environment. Humans and animals with continuous low-level exposure to DDT will accumulate it in their fat over time. Once animals die, the DDT from their bodies will be taken into the bodies of predators, or it will return to the environment for exposure to other living organisms, continuing the cycle of exposure, accumulation, and minimal degradation.

847. *Explain the difference between active transport and facilitated diffusion.*

Active transport involves a carrier that is specific for a chemical structure, and which can be competitively blocked by other chemicals. It requires energy, and can move molecules against a concentration or electrochemical gradient. It can be saturated at high substrate concentration, and the process can be blocked by inhibitors that can interfere with energy production. Facilitated diffusion involves a carrier that does not require energy, which can be saturated, and which cannot move molecules against a concentration or electrochemical gradient.

848. *Explain why weak organic acids are better absorbed through the stomach if total surface area is not considered.*

Non-ionized weak organic acids have much better lipid solubility and ability to penetrate cell membranes than the ionized form. According to the Henderson-Hasselbalch equation, at the low pH of the stomach, weak acids are much more present in the un-ionized form compared to the ionized form.

849. *Explain the different factors that determine the rate of absorption of gases in the lung.*

For gases that are poorly soluble in blood, the rate of absorption is considered perfusion-limited, and is dependent on blood flow through the lungs. For gases that are highly soluble in blood, the rate of absorption is considered ventilation-limited, and is dependent on the minute ventilation (rate and volume of respiration).

850. *Explain the anatomic and physiologic aspects of the blood-brain barrier.*

Anatomically, the capillary endothelial cells are close together with few pores, and they are surrounded by the cell processes of astrocytes. Physiologically, there are many active and facilitated transporters that can transport some chemicals out of endothelial cells back into the blood.

851. *Explain why sodium bicarbonate is an antidote for an overdose of phenobarbital.*

Phenobarbital is a weak organic acid. After consumption of sodium bicarbonate, the homeostatic mechanisms of the human body will keep the pH of blood and tissues constant by trapping bicarbonate ion in the renal tubules and raising the pH of urine to an alkaline level. At this high tubular pH, most phenobarbital will be ionized and will not be able to be reabsorbed back through the tubules. Thus, alkalinization of urine will increase the renal excretion of phenobarbital compared to an acidic urine, effectively removing phenobarbital from the body.

BIOTRANSFORMATION

852. *Explain why biotransformation enzymes evolved to convert toxicants into water-soluble chemicals to expedite their removal from the body.*

Our human ancestors were continuously exposed to unknown toxic substances as they explored their environments and tested new food sources. Many of these substances were chemically classified as alkaloids, which are lipid soluble. To remove these and other toxic substances from the body, a mechanism had to be established in which the lipid soluble compounds could not accumulate in in the lipid parts of the cells. The major routes of excretion for chemicals from the body are either through the kidney into the urine, or through the bile into the feces. To prevent chemicals from being reabsorbed in the tubules of the kidney, or the intestinal walls, they had to be made more polar and water soluble. Thus, biotransformation enzymes involved which convert lipid soluble nonpolar chemicals into water-soluble polar chemicals that can more readily be excreted in the urine and bile, so that they are permanently eliminated from the body.

853. Explain the process of enzyme induction.

Enzyme induction is a process by which a chemical can increase the activity of an enzyme by increasing the expression of the gene coding for that enzyme. With respect to drug metabolizing enzymes, one drug or chemical can increase the activity of an enzyme that metabolizes a variety of drugs. The inducing drug does not have to be metabolized by the enzyme that is induced. This process can produce clinically relevant drug-drug interactions. An inducing drug will cause an increase in the metabolic elimination of another substrate drug, thereby causing a decrease in the serum level of the substrate drug with a possible decrease in clinical response.

854. *Explain the process of enzyme inhibition and briefly describe three types.*

A chemical is classified as an enzyme inhibitor if it interacts with an enzyme and decreases its activity. A competitive inhibitor competes with the substrate for binding to the active site. A non-competitive inhibitor will bind to the enzyme and prevent the enzyme from completing the reaction. It can bind to the enzyme even when the substrate is already bound. A suicide inhibitor forms an irreversible chemical bond to the active site of the enzyme. Enzyme inhibitors can be drugs that produce clinically relevant drug-drug interactions by decreasing the metabolic elimination of a substrate drug, resulting in increased serum levels, and a possible increased clinical response or toxicity.

855. *Explain the significance of genetic polymorphisms in drug metabolism and name three cytochrome P-450s that exhibit genetic polymorphisms.*

Genetic polymorphisms in P-450 result in certain individuals being slower or faster metabolizers of drugs and chemicals, resulting in different levels of parent drugs and metabolites compared to individuals without the polymorphism. Examples are: CYP 2D6, CYP 2C9, CYP 2C19.

856. *Name some social factors and disease states that affect drug metabolism.*

Increased metabolism: cigarette smoking, chronic alcohol use, eating charcoal broiled meats Decreased metabolism: drinking grapefruit juice, infections, inflammation, cirrhosis

857. *Name the six conjugation reactions and the involved enzymes.*

Glucuronidation: UDP-glucuronyltransferase
Sulfonation: sulfotransferase
Methylation: methyltransferase
Acetylation: acetyltransferase
Glutathione conjugation: glutathione transferase
Amino acid conjugation: acetyl-CoA: amino acid N-acyltransferase

TOXICOKINETICS

858. Explain the difference between first-order kinetics and zero order kinetics.

In first-order kinetics, the rate of disappearance of the chemical is proportional to the concentration of chemical. This process has a concept called half-life, which is the time it takes for the blood or plasma concentration of the drug or toxicant to fall by 50%. Many biotransformation reactions for drugs and chemicals follow first-order kinetics. In zero order kinetics, a constant amount of chemical is eliminated from the body per unit time. The classic example of this is the elimination of ethanol from the human body, which is done at a rate of approximately 18 mg per deciliter of blood per hour. In overdose situations, many drugs and toxicants will shift from first-order kinetics to zero order kinetics.

859. *What is the concentration of 70 mg of a drug given intravenously with a volume of distribution of 2L/kg in the body of a 70kg man?*

Assume all 70 mg is completely absorbed intravenously
Volume of distribution is 70 kg x 2L/kg = 140 L
Drug concentration = 70 mg/140 L = 0.5 mg/L

860. *What are two plasma proteins that bind drugs?*

Albumin-usually binds acidic drugs
Alpha-1-acid glycoprotein-usually binds basic drugs

861. *In a two-compartment intravenous pharmacokinetic model, describe the distribution phase and elimination phase.*

The distribution phase is the time when the chemical leaves the plasma and is distributed to the body tissues. The elimination phase is the time when the drug in the blood and tissues is removed from the body, most commonly by excretion in the urine or biotransformation in the liver and other organs.

MECHANISMS OF TOXICITY

862. *Explain the difference between apoptosis and necrosis.*

Apoptosis or programmed cell death is an orderly process by which a cell destroys itself in response to certain stimuli such as toxicants or diseases. Apoptosis requires energy, and involves a controlled series of biochemical events. There is cell shrinkage and DNA fragmentation, without an inflammatory response. Insufficient apoptosis can promote the development of cancer, and exaggerated apoptosis may lead to neurodegenerative diseases. Necrosis or accidental cell death involves cell swelling and cell membrane rupture, frequently followed by an inflammatory response. Unlike apoptosis, which can involve individual cells, necrosis usually occurs in multiple adjacent cells, or large regions of tissue. Necrosis is a typical response to a large amount of toxicant.

863. *Describe all the stages from toxicant exposure to toxicity at the cellular level.*

An organism is usually exposed to a toxicant either through the skin, gastrointestinal tract, respiratory tract, or placenta. Sometimes exposure can take place through bites or human injection. Once exposed, the toxicant is absorbed into the body and distributed away from the site of absorption into the entire body. Certain target organs may be particularly vulnerable to the toxicant due to selective accumulation or to selective metabolism into a more toxic substance known as the ultimate toxicant. This final chemical will damage proteins, lipids and nucleic acids resulting in toxicity by various mechanisms, such as interference with gene expression, interference with cellular activity, depletion of ATP, increasing intracellular calcium, and mitochondrial dysfunction.

864. *Explain how oxygen can be essential to a human organism and toxic at the same time.*

Molecular oxygen is essential for the process of oxidative phosphorylation by which ATP is produced in mitochondria. However, molecular oxygen can also gain energy and convert to a more reactive form called singlet oxygen. Molecular oxygen can also be reduced by a series of reactions and become the reactive molecules: superoxide anion radical, hydrogen peroxide, and hydroxyl radical. Collectively, all these new forms of reactive oxygen are called reactive oxygen species (ROS). They can cause damage to DNA, proteins, and lipids.

865. *Explain how cyanide toxicity can occur in the home, and the mechanism of cyanide toxicity.*

Hydrogen cyanide gas can be produced in the home when polyurethane plastics catch fire. Cyanide anion binds to the terminal cytochrome c oxidase in the electron transport chain, causing a rapid reduction of intracellular ATP production, with resultant cell death.

866. *Briefly describe the role of calcium ion in normal physiology and in toxic conditions.*

Calcium ion is involved in important physiologic processes such as signaling, enzyme activation and being a second messenger. The concentration of extracellular calcium is approximately 10,000 times higher than intracellular calcium. This large concentration gradient is sustained by ATP dependent calcium pumps. Toxicants can interfere with the concentration gradient of calcium and cause a fast influx of calcium into the cell, leading to cell injury, apoptosis, or necrosis.

867. *List four nuclear receptors and chemicals that bind to them potentially leading to a toxic response.*

Aryl hydrocarbon receptor – TCDD
Estrogen receptor – nonylphenol
Androgen receptor – DDT metabolite
Peroxisome proliferator-activated receptor – phthalate plasticizers

TESTING METHODS

868. *Briefly describe the five phases of clinical drug research.*

Phase 0: Pre-clinical testing in laboratory animals for pharmacology, toxicology and formulation development.

Phase 1: Testing in normal healthy volunteers for safety and pharmacokinetics.

Phase 2: Testing in small numbers of patients for safety and efficacy.

Phase 3: Testing in thousands of patients for safety and efficacy.

Phase 4: Continued testing after drug is FDA approved.

869. *List two non-animal toxicology testing methods that may be able to replace traditional animal testing.*

In vitro cell and tissue cultures
In silico (computer) simulations

CARCINOGENESIS/MUTAGENESIS

870. *Explain the three stages of carcinogenesis.*

The first stage or initiation involves the mutation of DNA by a chemical, virus, or radiation. If this mutated cell is not repaired, it can be involved in the second stage or promotion. In this stage, the mutated cell undergoes a clonal proliferation in the presence of a promoter such as a hormone. In the final stage or progression, the cells in the clonal proliferation are subjected to more mutations and are transformed into a true cancer cell that is capable of un-regulated growth, invasiveness, and distant spread to other organs and tissues.

871. *Explain the difference between a benign and malignant tumor.*

A benign tumor is made up of cells that proliferate faster than nor-mal cells, but are usually surrounded by a capsule, and do not in-vade into other tissues. A malignant tumor is composed of grossly abnormal cells, that rapidly proliferate and invade locally. They will eventually spread to other organs and tissues, resulting in the death of the organism.

872. *Describe the Ames test.*

A mutated version of the bacteria Salmonella typhimurium (which cannot grow unless histidine is added to the culture) is used for the test. In the presence of mutagenic chemicals, some mutated bacteria will convert back to a form that does not need external histidine. The mutated bacteria are plated with a nutrient medium that does not contain histidine. When a test chemical is added, if any colonies form, the chemical is considered a mutagen.

873. *Explain the threshold and non-threshold models for carcinogenesis.*

The non-threshold model assumes cancer can be produced by one molecule of a carcinogen. The non-threshold model assumes that at low levels of carcinogen exposure, mechanisms of DNA repair, detoxication, and immune destruction will prevent the development of cancer up to a certain threshold exposure.

874. *Explain how a chemical can be negative in the Ames test and still be classified as a carcinogen.*

The Ames test shows whether a chemical can damage DNA. Carcinogens which are promoters act by non-mutagenic mechanisms and would be negative in the Ames test. Promoters can act by stimulating cell growth, inhibiting apoptosis, inhibiting DNA repair, and hindering cell to cell communication.

875. *Explain why metabolic activation may be necessary in the Ames test.*

Many carcinogens need to be transformed to mutagenic metabolites by cytochrome P-450s. To "metabolically activate" these procarcinogens to true carcinogens, a fraction of liver homogenate that contains microsomes (cytochrome P-450) called S9 is added to the test mixture.

876. *Explain the role of DNA methylation in the development of cancer.*

DNA methylation regulates gene transcription. Hypermethylation generally leads to a suppressing of gene activity. If this happens to tumor suppressor genes, there is increased risk of cancer. Hypomethylation of DNA can lead to lead to increased gene expression. This process has also been linked to increased cancer risk.

DEVELOPMENTAL AND REPRODUCTIVE TOXICOLOGY

877. *Describe the three critical periods of teratogenesis.*

During the fertilization to gastrula stage, exposure usually result in complete survival or death. Exposures during the period of organogenesis can result in malformations of organ systems. Exposures during the fetal period can lead to growth retardation and effects on the central nervous system

878. *Describe the proposed mechanism of teratogenicity for thalidomide.*

Thalidomide was a drug prescribed during the late 1950s and early 1960s to relieve the morning sickness of pregnancy. It was associated with severe shortening of the limbs and other major birth defects. It has a number of effects on cellular physiology, however the leading theory for its teratogenicity is that it inhibits the formation of new blood vessels in the embryo (angiogenesis inhibitor).

879. *Name three commonly prescribed drugs and their associated teratogenicity.*

Phenytoin (anti-seizure) – craniofacial abnormalities, limb defects, growth deficiency, mental retardation
Valproic acid (anti-seizure) – spina bifida
Isotretinoin (anti-acne) – malformations of ears, heart, brain, thymus

880. *Name a class of antihypertensive drug that is an exception in that it causes major organ dysfunction during third trimester exposure.*

Angiotensin converting enzyme (ACE) inhibitors and angiotensin receptor blockers (ARB) when administered during the third trimester have been associated with hypocalvaria, pulmonary hypoplasia, and major kidney abnormalities that can lead to fetal death.

881. *Describe the fetal-alcohol syndrome.*

There is no safe time or safe amount of alcohol to drink during pregnancy. Women who drink while pregnant are at risk for having children with a spectrum of physical, psychological and behavior problems. The most severe manifestation is called the fetal alcohol syndrome and consists of growth retardation, craniofacial abnormalities, impaired psychomotor and intellectual development, and other abnormalities.

882. *Describe the toxic effects of maternal diethylstilbestrol (DES) use on male and female offspring.*

DES was used to treat threatened miscarriage. Daughters of exposed mothers had a high incidence of reproductive tract abnormalities and a rare cancer know as clear cell adenocarcinoma of the vagina. Sons of exposed mothers also have a higher risk of urogenital abnormalities and testicular cancer.

IMMUNE SYSTEM TOXICOLOGY

883. *Explain autoimmunity, and describe two ways toxicants can trigger autoimmunity.*

Autoimmunity is when the body's own antibodies cause disease by attacking tissues that should be considered "self". Toxicants may damage tissues and produce an abnormal condition that may be recognized by the immune system as "non-self" with resultant immune attack. Also, toxicants may chemically resemble tissue surface molecules such that an immune response against the toxicant results in an attack on the bystander tissue.

884. *Name four drugs that cause autoimmune disease.*

Halothane – hepatitis
Quinine – thrombocytopenia
Amoxicillin – hemolytic anemia
Hydralazine – systemic lupus erythematosus

885. *Give an example of a toxicant that can cause a type I allergic reaction.*

A type I allergic reaction is an antigen – IgE antibody reaction that triggers the release of histamine, serotonin, chemokines and other inflammatory mediators that can produce asthma, urticaria and anaphylaxis. Toluene diisocyanate is an industrial chemical that can induce a type I allergic response.

886. *Name some toxicants that elicit a type IV allergic response.*

A type IV allergic response is mediated by activation of T cells. This reaction on the skin is the commonly seen contact dermatitis due to poison ivy, poison oak, nickel, and latex. Beryllium can produce a type IV reaction in the lung.

887. *Define immunosuppression and name some toxicants associated with it.*

Immunosuppression is a decrease in response of one or all the components of the immune system. It can lead to increased susceptibility to infections and cancer. TCDD, PCBs, DDT, and lead are examples of toxicants that cause immunosuppression in laboratory animals.

888. *Name some drugs that elicit a type III allergic response.*

A type III allergic response is the deposition of antigen-antibody complexes in tissues or blood vessel walls with resultant inflammation. Antibiotics, snake anti-venom, monoclonal antibodies, and gold are examples of causative agents.

HEMATOLOGIC TOXICOLOGY

889. *Describe hemolytic anemia and give examples of drugs/toxicants that cause it.*

Drugs/toxicants can act as haptens and cause the immune system to produce antibodies against red cells leading to their premature destruction. This mechanism is called hemolytic anemia. Penicillin, methyldopa and arsine can cause this process.

890. *Describe iron deficiency anemia and name a class of drugs associated with it.*

When there is not enough iron in the body to efficiency produce normal red cells, the red cells created are fewer and smaller. Iron deficiency from diet is rare in the developed world, but is commonly caused by blood loss. Non-steroidal anti-inflammatory drugs can cause stomach erosions and ulcers leading to asymptomatic or overt bleeding. If bleeding is significant, eventually iron deficiency anemia will develop.

891. *Describe megaloblastic anemia and a common drug/toxicant associated with it.*

In megaloblastic anemias, red cells are larger than normal due to defective DNA synthesis. This causes the cell to grow and not divide, leading to fewer but larger cells. Drugs that interfere with folate metabolism or dietary intake such as methotrexate and ethanol are causative.

892. *Describe the anemia of bone marrow depression and give an example of a causative agent.*

In bone marrow depression or aplastic anemia, the production of all hematologic cells (red cells, white cells, platelets) is suppressed at the precursor level. Sometimes, only the red cell line is involved, and this is called pure red cell aplasia. Benzene has been implicated in producing aplastic anemia.

893. *Explain why carbon monoxide poisoning produces a "cherry red cyanosis".*

Carbon dioxide binds to hemoglobin to form carboxyhemoglobin which is a brighter red compared to the color of normal oxygenated hemoglobin. In severe carbon monoxide poisonings, the skin can appear a bright red color as the patient is dying from hypoxia.

894. *Describe methemoglobinemia, some toxicants that are causative, and the antidote.*

Methemoglobin is produced when the iron in hemoglobin is oxidized to the ferric state. It causes a shift in the oxygen-hemoglobin dissociation curve to the left and a resultant decreased ability of oxygen to be released to the tissues. It can be caused by consuming large amounts of nitrates and nitrites in foods, and by exposure to nitrobenzene or benzocaine. Methylene blue, the antidote works by reducing the ferric ion in hemoglobin back to ferrous ion.

HEPATIC TOXICOLOGY

895. *Describe fatty liver and list three drugs/toxicants that are causative?*

Fatty liver or steatosis is when the liver is composed of more than 5% lipid by weight. It can occur from increased production of triglycerides, or impaired release of triglycerides from the hepatocyte into the blood. Ethanol, tetracycline, and phosphorus are causative.

896. *Describe cholestasis and list three drugs/toxicants that are causative?*

Cholestasis is the inability of the liver to efficiently excrete bile. The bile backs up into the liver and causes damage. Chlorpromazine, anabolic and estrogenic steroids, and alpha-naphthylisocyanate are causative.

897. *Describe hepatic necrosis and list three drugs/toxicants that are causative.*

Hepatic necrosis is irreversible hepatocyte injury leading to the death of hepatocytes with rupture of the cell membrane. The release of inflammatory mediators can cause neighboring normal cells to be involved. Acetaminophen, bromobenzene, and carbon tetrachloride are causative.

898. *Describe cirrhosis and list two drugs/toxicants that are causative.*

Cirrhosis or liver fibrosis is the deposition of collagen (scar tissue) throughout the liver. At advanced stages, there is interference with hepatic blood flow and altered physiology and biochemistry. Chronic ethanol use and methotrexate are causative.

899. *Describe drug/toxicant induced hepatitis and list two causative agents.*

Drug/toxicant induced hepatitis is inflammation of the liver that resembles viral hepatitis. Isoniazid (anti-tuberculosis) and halothane (anesthetic) are causative.

900. *List three forms of hepatic cancer and their causative agents.*

Hepatocellular carcinoma – possibly chronic androgen abuse
Angiosarcoma – vinyl chloride
Cholangiocarcinoma – radioactive thorium dioxide (Thorotrast)

RENAL TOXICOLOGY

901. *Explain the role of the glomerulus and list some toxicants* that affect it.

The glomerulus receives blood under pressure and acts to produce an ultrafiltrate of plasma. Large molecules over 70,000 MW are not filtered, whereas smaller molecules enter Bowman's capsule and flow into the proximal convoluted tubule and distil parts of the nephron. Gold, lead, and puromycin can damage the glomerulus.

902. *Explain the role of the proximal convoluted tubule and list some toxicants that affect it.*

The proximal convoluted tubule reabsorbs sodium, water, and all other essential electrolytes, along with glucose, amino acids, small proteins, and citric acid cycle intermediates. It also excretes weak organic anions and cations into the tubular fluid. Aminoglycoside antibiotics, carbon tetrachloride, and chloroform are toxic to the proximal convoluted tubule.

903. *Briefly describe the functions of the kidney not involved in urine production.*

The kidney produces renin, which helps to regulate blood pressure through the renin-angiotensin-aldosterone system. It converts an inactive form of vitamin D to an active form which is important in calcium homeostasis. It helps to make erythropoietin which stimulates the production of red blood cells by the bone marrow.

904. *Briefly describe the role of the loop of Henle and distil convoluted tubule, and name a drug class associated with injury to this region.*

Filtrate that passes through the loop of Henle and distil convoluted tubule undergoes further reabsorption of electrolytes and water with a reduction in volume. Long term use of some non-steroidal anti-inflammatory drugs such as aspirin, ibuprofen, acetaminophen, and phenacetin (alone or in combination) can cause damage to this area of the kidney. The condition is called analgesic nephropathy.

905. *Briefly describe the role of the collecting duct and name a toxicant to this area.*

The collecting duct functions to produce a concentrated or dilute urine through the action of antidiuretic hormone (ADH). In the absence of ADH, no significant additional concentration of urine will occur. If ADH is present, the urine will be further concentrated. Methoxyflurane (anesthetic) can be toxic to this region by possible blocking the action of ADH on the collecting duct.

906. *Describe obstructive uropathy and name three causative agents.*

Obstructive uropathy occurs when toxicants precipitate out of tubular fluid or urine in the ureter. The obstruction causes a back pressure which damages renal cells behind the obstruction. The common name for the process on a large scale is "kidney stone formation". Ethylene glycol (through the formation of oxalic acid) and melamine are causative.

907. *Briefly discuss the susceptibility of the kidney to toxicant injury, and its capacity for repair.*

The renal cells achieve higher concentrations of toxicants than most other organs. This is due to high renal blood flow, presence of cytochrome p-450 (ability to directly form toxic metabolites), and tubular concentrating ability. These factors make the kidney particularly vulnerable to toxicant induced injury. In contrast, the kidney has an exceptional capacity for compensation and repair. However, long term compensatory mechanisms may contribute to chronic renal failure.

ENDOCRINE TOXICOLOGY

908. *Describe the toxic effects of glucocorticoids.*

In excess, glucocorticoids can cause a number of adverse effects. Some common ones are depressed immune function, impaired wound healing, acne, muscle weakness, edema, mental depression, and osteoporosis. Chronic use of high doses of glucocorticoids will depress ACTH secretion by the pituitary, leading to adrenal insufficiency if the glucocorticoids are suddenly stopped or severely tapered.

909. *Describe some of the toxic effects of chronic androgen use in athletes or body builders.*

Anabolic steroid use is associated with increased risk of cardiovascular disease, central nervous system disease (aggression, mood changes, psychosis), acne, benign liver tumors, and infertility.

910. *Describe some toxic effects of estrogen therapy.*

Common adverse effects of estrogens include headache, nausea, irregular vaginal bleeding, bloating, and breast pain. Some serious adverse effects reported include blood clots in the legs and certain cancers.

911. *Describe the signs and symptoms of hypothyroidism and hyperthyroidism, and name some causative drugs/toxicants.*

Some signs and symptoms of hypothyroidism include weight gain, fatigue, hair loss, constipation, cold intolerance, muscle cramps, and slow heart rate. Some signs and symptoms of hyperthyroidism include tremor, diarrhea, rapid heart rate, arrhythmias, weight loss and insomnia. Drug/toxicant induced hyperthyroidism is rare, but can be caused by iodine and amiodarone. Hypothyroidism can be caused by agents listed in the question below, and possibly by polycyclic halogenated hydrocarbons.

912. *Name some agents that disrupt thyroid hormone synthesis.*

Anion inhibitors like thiocyanate anion and perchlorate anion can competitively block the iodide transport system which brings iodide into the thyroid from the blood against a concentration gradient. Drugs like methimazole and propylthiouracil inhibit the thyroperoxidase enzyme which: 1) oxidizes iodide to iodine which then combines with tyrosine to form monoiodotyrosine (MIT) and diiodotyrosine (DIT); 2) couples DIT and MIT to form T3 or DIT and DIT to form T4.

TOXICOLOGY OF THE EYE

913. *Explain why alkali exposure to the cornea is more toxic than acid exposure.*

Both strong acids and strong alkalis can cause severe damage to the cornea. The extent of damage is related to the concentration of offending agent and duration of exposure. Alkalis are particularly toxic because they penetrate the cornea rapidly and they can have both an acute phase of toxicity followed by a second phase of corneal ulceration weeks later.

914. *Explain how systemic absorption of a chemical that is splashed or intentionally placed in the eye can occur.*

Chemicals in contact with the eye will first be washed away by tears. Any remaining chemical will enter the vascularized conjunctiva and be absorbed into the blood. Also, some of the chemical can pass through the nasolacrimal duct into the digestive tract and be absorbed.

915. *List some drugs and toxicants bound to intraocular melanin.*

Melanin is found in the iris, ciliary body, retinal pigmented epithelium, and uveal tract. Heavy metals such as lead, polycyclic aromatic hydrocarbons, and the drugs atropine and chloroquine can bind to melanin in high concentrations

916. Define cataract and list two drug classes associated with its occurrence.

A cataract is an opacification in the lens of the eye that can result in decreased vision. It is usually associated with increased age, however, they have been associated with the chronic use of corticosteroids and phenothiazines (antipsychotic drug).

917. Name three reasons why the retina is particularly sensitive to toxicants.

1) high rate of mitochondrial oxidative phosphorylation
2) high blood flow
3) the potential for phototoxicity of certain chemicals

918. Discuss drug metabolizing enzymes in the eye.

The tears, cornea, iris, lens, retina, and choroid of various experimental animals are capable of drug metabolism. Varying types of phase I and phase II enzymes are present in these components. Sine the eye has external contact with many chemicals, and has the potential for phototoxicity, the presence of glutathione detoxifying enzymes is very important.

TOXICOLOGY OF SKIN

919. *Discuss the skin as a barrier to toxicant absorption.*

The outer stratum corneum is composed of dead cells and provides the most effective barrier against toxicants. Loss of integrity of the stratum corneum by psoriasis or abrasions will significantly increase the permeability of toxicants. Once in the living layer of epidermis below the stratum corneum, both lipid soluble and water-soluble chemicals can be easily absorbed into the blood, and be distributed systemically.

920. *Explain the difference between photo-allergy and photo-toxicity.*

Photo-toxicity can occur after a single exposure, and requires the photochemical absorption of energy from light, and subsequent production of toxic free radicals. A photo-allergic reaction requires light to interact with a chemical to produce a hapten, which then elicits the classic immune response. The amount of reacting chemical is usually lower in a photo-allergic reaction, and a time delay between exposures is necessary.

921. *Discuss the biotransformation ability of the skin.*

The skin contains both phase I and phase II biotransformation enzymes. It can perform both detoxication and metabolic activation of chemicals into sensitizers or carcinogens.

922. *Discuss the difference between irritant dermatitis and allergic contact dermatitis.*

Irritant dermatitis is a direct toxic reaction of a chemical with the skin that does not involve the immune system. The severity of the reaction is directly exposure related. Allergic contact dermatitis requires initial sensitization to an antigenic chemical, and repeat exposure to elicit the response.

923. *Describe toxic epidermal necrolysis and some causative drugs.*

Toxic epidermal necrolysis is the most severe skin reaction caused by drugs and chemicals. It involves the complete necrosis of the epidermis and resembles a burn. The epidermis sloughs off, and only the dermis remains as a very compromised barrier to loss of fluids and electrolytes. The antiepileptic drugs phenytoin and carbamazepine are causative.

924. *Discuss the roles of UV-A, UV-B, and UV-C ultraviolet radiation in the genesis of skin cancer.*

UV-C radiation is the shortest wavelength and the most damaging to skin. However, it is absorbed by the atmosphere and does not reach the surface of the earth. UV-B radiation is also mostly absorbed by the atmosphere, however, the radiation that does reach the earth, is responsible for the development of melanoma and non-melanoma skin cancers. Ninety-five percent of the UV radiation reaching the earth's surface is the long wavelength UV-A. Recent studies suggest that it may also contribute to the development of skin cancer.

NEUROTOXICOLOGY

925. Name the cell types in the nervous system and their function.

Neurons carry electrical messages between the brain and organs of the body. Astrocytes are "star shaped" cells that provide structure and are involved in metabolism and the regulation of neuronal transmission in the brain. Oligodendrocytes synthesize myelin in the central nervous system, and Schwann cells synthesize myelin in the peripheral nervous system.

926. *Discuss the energy need of the nervous system.*

Neurons consume large amounts of energy to maintain and recreate ion gradients, interact with neurotransmitters, provide active transport into the brain, conduct axonal transport, and perform other functions. Neurons rely on aerobic glycolysis as a continual source of energy. They are particularly vulnerable to toxicants that interfere with ATP production or create a state of hypoxia or glucose deficiency.

927. *Describe axonopathy and name some toxicants that are causative.*

The damage in an axonopathy occurs initially only to the axon, and not the cell body. However, with time, damage can progress to the entire neuron. Axonopathies frequently occur in the peripheral nervous system, and can be reversible there. However, regeneration of axons does not occur in the central nervous system. Acrylamide and a metabolite of n-hexane are causative.

928. *Describe the "Ginger Jake" mass poisoning.*

During Prohibition, a toxic organophosphate known as triortho-cresyl phosphate was added to tonics in place of ginger. Many thousands of people developed an axonopathy and neurological symptoms after exposure. Some were left with permanent paralysis.

929. Describe neuronopathy and name some toxicants that are causative.

A neuronopathy is damage to the nerve cell body, resulting in dysfunction or death. Effects on the brain can produce many neurological events such as seizures, dementia, and coma. Cyanide, methyl mercury, lead, and carbon monoxide are examples of causative agents.

930. *Describe a myelinopathy and name some toxicants that are causative.*

A myelinopathy occurs when there is selective damage to the myelin covering of central and peripheral nerves. Nerve conduction is slowed or completely halted, with resulting neurological symptoms. Hexachlorophene and triethyltin are causative.

931. *Name some naturally occurring toxins and the neurotransmitters that they affect.*

Ergot alkaloids – alpha adrenergic receptors
Picrotoxin – GABA receptors
Cocaine – dopamine, serotonin, norepinephrine
Kainic acid – glutamate
Strychnine – glycine

932. *Discuss the role of MPTP in toxicant induced Parkinson's disease.*

MPTP is a contaminant of the synthesis of the opioid MPPP. It can cross the blood-brain barrier and be metabolized to MPP+ which accumulates in dopaminergic neurons and causes damage. The result is a syndrome that resembles naturally occurring Parkinson's disease.

933. *Explain why the developing nervous system is particularly vulnerable to toxicants.*

The nervous system develops and matures during the embryonic, fetal, and postnatal periods. During this long time span, there is an opportunity for toxicants to exert a variety of effects on structure and function. The incomplete development of the blood-brain barrier also contributes to the vulnerability.

CARDIOVASCULAR TOXICOLOGY

934. *Explain why the QT interval is important in cardiac toxicology.*

The QT interval represents the period of cardiac muscle cell depolarization and repolarization. When prolonged, there is abnormal activity of the sodium and potassium channels which can lead to life threatening arrhythmias. There is an inherited form of QT prolongation and an acquired form induced by drugs such as fluoroquinolone antibiotics, tricyclic antidepressants, and quinidine. There is greater susceptibility to the arrhythmogenic effects of QT prolonging drugs in overdose situations.

935. *Explain the pathogenesis of cardiomyopathy, and some drugs and toxicants that are causative.*

When some myocytes are damaged, the remaining myocytes undergo hypertrophy to compensate. Sometimes this hypertrophy is accompanied by fibrosis. With time, compensation fails, and the pumping ability of the heart decreases. This pathologic condition is called cardiomyopathy, and the clinical result is called congestive heart failure. Recent research suggests that some damage can be reversed through the use of stem cells. Alcohol, cobalt, and the anticancer drug doxorubicin are causative.

936. *Explain the toxicity of digitalis glycosides on the heart.*

Digitalis is present in the foxglove plant. It inhibits Na+/K+ ATPase which results in an increase in intracellular sodium and a reduction of intracellular potassium. It also reduces calcium egress from the cells, and increases the force of contraction of the heart. With toxicity, the electrolyte imbalance significantly interferes with the resting membrane potential and leads to life-threatening arrhythmias.

937. *Explain why some workers exposed to nitroglycerin during the week have died during the weekend.*

Nitroglycerin can dilate coronary arteries. During the week, the workers experience a certain degree of coronary blood flow in the presence of nitroglycerin. Because of its short half-life, the nitroglycerin effects are gone on the weekend. Some workers whose coronary blood flow was dependent on nitroglycerin, would then be vulnerable to myocardial ischemia, and sudden death.

938. *Name some toxicants which may accelerate atherosclerosis with chronic exposure.*

Carbon disulfide, nanoparticle air pollution, cocaine, carbon monoxide.

939. *Name some toxins which damage the endothelial cells of capillaries and cause bleeding.*

Snake venom toxin, ebola virus glycoprotein

RESPIRATORY TOXICOLOGY

940. *Describe the ways the respiratory system protects itself from particle toxicants.*

Particles are trapped and moved away from the lung by mucus and cilia present in the upper airway. Particles from this "mucociliary escalator" can then be eliminated by swallowing. Particles reaching the lower portions of the lungs are engulfed by phagocytic macrophages which then ride the mucociliary escalator, and are removed.

941. *Describe the penetration of gases into the lung based on water solubility.*

Highly water-soluble gases like sulfur dioxide dissolve in the mucus of the nose and upper airway, and usually do not reach the lung. Water insoluble gases like ozone can reach the small bronchioles and alveoli and cause toxicity.

942. *Describe the etiology of lung fibrosis and some causative agents.*

Chronic exposure to dusts creates diseases called pneumoconiosis. Dust particles settle in the alveoli, and are engulfed by macrophages. However, the macrophages, are inefficient in particle removal, and inflammatory mediators are released during the process, which stimulates fibroblasts and collagen deposition. Silica dust, coal dust, and asbestos are causative.

943. *Describe the proposed etiology of emphysema.*

Emphysema is thought to result from increased lung proteinase activity or decreased lung anti-proteinase activity. The result is destruction of alveoli walls, enlargement of air spaces, loss of elasticity, air trapping, and impaired gas exchange. Cigarette smoking is the most common etiologic factor, however, in some countries, indoor air pollution from poorly ventilated cooking fires is the principal cause.

944. *Describe hypersensitivity pneumonitis.*

Hypersensitivity pneumonitis is an immune reaction that occurs in the alveoli after repetitive exposure to organic dusts such as moldy hay. The disease can be acute, sub-acute, or chronic, and is thought to involve both type III and type IV hypersensitivity.

945. *Name some toxicants associated with human lung cancer.*
Cigarette smoke (active and passive), radon, asbestos, arsenic, air pollution, diesel exhaust

TOXICOLOGY OF METALS
946. *Name some signs and symptoms of acute and chronic arsenic toxicity.*

After acute ingestion, arsenic can cause fever, abdominal pain, vomiting, diarrhea, encephalopathy, peripheral neuropathy, hematologic abnormalities, cardiac arrhythmias and cardiac failure. Chronic exposure can cause skin and possibly other cancers, liver disease, cardiovascular disease, and peripheral neuropathy.

947. *Describe metal fume fever.*

Metal fume fever occurs after exposure to chemicals present in the fumes of heated metals. Oxides of zinc, aluminum, and magnesium are some causative chemicals. Symptoms begin with a metallic taste, and are similar to the flu. Resolution usually occurs within 1 to 2 days.

948. *Describe the toxic effects of cadmium on three major target organs.*

Cadmium can cause soft bones (osteomalacia), and demineralized bones (osteoporosis). It damages the glomeruli and tubules of the kidney leading to renal failure. Some studies have shown that long -term cadmium inhalation is associated with obstructive lung disease.

949. *Contrast the toxicity of organic arsenic and organic mercury.*

Organic arsenic chemicals (like those present in seafood) are less toxic than inorganic arsenic chemicals (like those present in contaminated drinking water). In contrast, organic mercury is extremely neurotoxic.

950. *Comment on the toxicity of nickel carbonyl.*

Nickel carbonyl $Ni(CO)_4$ is one of the most toxic industrial chemicals. It is a flammable liquid that can auto-ignite. It is rapidly absorbed through the skin or by inhalation. Toxicity after acute exposure involves the respiratory and neurologic systems

951. *What are metallothioneins?*

Metallothioneins are intracellular binding proteins that play an important role in binding essential and toxic metals. Their concentrations can be increased (induced) by exposure to metals and pathologic conditions. Dysfunction of metallothioneins have been implicated in disease.

TOXICITY OF PESTICIDES

952. *Explain the mechanism of action of organophosphorous insecticides and their toxicity.*

Organophosphorous insecticides inhibit the enzyme acetylcholinesterase resulting in muscarinic cholinergic symptoms of sweating and salivation, bronchoconstriction, diarrhea; and nicotinic cholinergic symptoms of muscle twitching and paralysis. Cholinergic stimulation of both receptors also leads to cardiovascular and central nervous system effects. Pralidoxime can be an antidote if given early, but with time inhibition of the enzyme becomes irreversible (aged) and new enzyme synthesis is necessary to restore enzyme activity back to normal.

953. *Explain the delayed toxic syndromes associated with organo-phosphorous insecticides.*

A delayed weakness of respiratory, facial, and neck muscles can occur 1 to 4 days after organophosphorous exposure. The symptoms seem to occur, at the end of the cholinergic period. A syndrome of organophosphorous induced delayed polyneuropathy (OPIDP) with sensory and motor loss to the extremities can occur 2 to 3 weeks after exposure.

954. *Explain the mechanism of action of pyrethrins.*

Pyrethrins interfere with the closing of voltage-gated sodium channels in insects. They have low mammalian toxicity

955. *Explain the mechanism of action of the organochlorine insecticide DDT.*

DDT prevents the closing of voltage-gated sodium channels similar to pyrethrins.

956. *Explain the mechanism of action of Lindane and cyclodienes.*

Lindane and cyclodienes block the opening of the inhibitory chloride channel. They oppose the action of the inhibitory neurotransmitter GABA.

957. *Explain the mechanism of action of dinitrophenols.*

Dinitrophenols acts to siphon protons away from the proton gradient that mitochondria use to produce ATP. Instead of storing chemical energy in ATP, dinitrophenol causes the energy to be lost as heat.

CHEMICAL AND SOLVENT TOXICOLOGY

958. Discuss the relationship between lipid solubility and central nervous system effects of solvents.

There is a direct relationship between lipid solubility of solvents and central nervous system depression. The degree of depression seems to be proportional to the length of carbon chains, number of double bonds, and number of halogen atoms.

959. Discuss the possible existence of a solvent-induced chronic encephalopathy.

Epidemiologic studies conducted on individuals with workplace exposure to high daily concentrations of a variety of solvents have suggested that a syndrome of chronic encephalopathy may exist. Impairments in memory, changes in mood and personality, and decline in intellectual function have been reported.

960. *In general, what is the effect of organic solvents on the heart.*

All organic solvents may cause the heart to be more sensitive to the arrhythmogenic effects of endogenous epinephrine. In animal models, halogenated hydrocarbons seem to be the most toxic class.

961. *Discuss the health effects of the aromatic hydrocarbons benzene and toluene.*

In addition to the central nervous system and cardiac effects mentioned above, benzene and toluene have some specific toxicities. Benzene is associated with bone marrow depression which can affect the production of all or some of the cellular elements of the blood. Benzene is also strongly implicated as a cause of leukemia. Toluene is associated with a variety of renal diseases.

962. *Explain why ethyl alcohol is an antidote for methyl alcohol and ethylene glycol poisoning.*

Ethyl alcohol, methyl alcohol, and ethylene glycol are all metabolized by the same enzyme. The metabolite of methyl alcohol is the toxicant (formic acid), and the metabolite of ethylene glycol is the toxicant (oxalic acid). Ethyl alcohol acts as an antidote by competitively blocking sites on the enzyme that convert methyl alcohol and ethylene glycol to their toxic metabolites. By delaying the conversion to the toxic metabolites, more of the parent compounds can be eliminated by the kidney or dialysis before conversion.

963. *Name some toxic components of gasoline.*

Benzene, toluene, naphthalene, n-hexane, methyl tertiary-butyl ether.

FOOD TOXICOLOGY

964. *What is a food additive?*

A food additive is a substance that would not be eaten by itself as a food, but is added to food in small amounts for the purpose of preservation, improving texture, color, consistency, or taste.

Example are food colors and artificial sweeteners.

965. *What is an indirect food additive.*

An indirect food additive is a substance that contaminates food by coming in contact with food during its processing, storage, or shipment. An example is plasticizer.

966. *What is a GRAS substance?*

Generally recognized as safe or "GRAS" is a food additive that is exempt from testing by the Food and Drug Administration because it has an extensive history of use in human foods without safety concerns. Examples are helium and acetic acid.

967. *What is a food contaminant?*

A food contaminant is a substance present in food that was not intentionally added. An example is pesticide residue.

968. *Name some molds that contaminate food and possible toxicities.*

Aflatoxin – liver cancer
Ochratoxin – renal toxic
Fumonisin – cancer, neural tube birth defects

969. *Name some foods that can interfere with biotransformation enzymes.*

Grapefruit and grapefruit juice, charcoal broiled meats, brussel sprouts

ECOTOXICOLOGY

970. *What are primary air pollutants and name the major classes.*

Primary air pollutants enter the atmosphere as the result of a natural or industrial activity. Major classes include the oxides of carbon, sulfur, and nitrogen, volatile hydrocarbons, heavy metals, and particulate matter.

971. *What are secondary air pollutants and name the major examples.*

Secondary air pollutants are synthesized from primary pollutants by photochemical reactions. Example are ozone, peroxy-acetyl nitrate, hydrogen peroxide, and aldehydes.

972. *Name the major greenhouse gases.*

Carbon dioxide, water vapor, methane, ozone, nitrous oxide.

973. *Describe the formation of acid rain and its toxic effects.*

Acid rain forms from the reaction of rain water with oxides of nitrogen and sulfur in the atmosphere. It has an adverse effect on soil, fish hatching, freshwater ecosystems, growth of some plants, and formation of limestone skeletons in corals.

974. *Name some potential toxic effects of plastic accumulation in the ocean.*

Many marine animals die from directing eating plastics. Indirectly, the plastics can concentrate organic toxicants like PCBs, and PAHs. These toxicants can enter lower forms of ocean life, and may eventually move all the way through the food chain to humans.

975. *Discuss ways to clean up oil spills.*

Skimming the oil off the surface, burning the oil on the surface of the water, and applying chemical dispersants that act like detergents which break the oil up into small droplets, are the principal ways to clean up an oil spill. The use of dispersants is controversial, as they can be toxic in themselves, and can spread the oil to uncontaminated areas. Some advocate doing nothing, and letting natural processes like the sun, wind and weather perform the cleanup. Research is being done to create genetically engineered microbes that are more efficient than naturally occurring microbes in consuming oil.

TOXIC PLANTS AND ANIMALS

976. *Name some plants that contain cardiac toxins.*

Foxglove, lily of the valley, squill, milkweed

977. *Name some plants that contain anticholinergic alkaloids.*

Nightshade, jimsonweed, henbane

978. *Name three toxic spiders that can be found in the United States.*

American funnel web spider, black widow, brown recluse

979. *Name two venom producing lizards.*

Gila monster, bearded lizard

980. *Name some excitatory amino acid agonists and the plants that contain them.*

.

Kainic acid – species of marine red algae
Domoic acid – species of marine green algae
Ibotenic acid – species of wild mushroom

TOXICOLOGY OF PRESCRIPTION AND OVER-THE-COUNTER MEDICATIONS

981. *Discuss the toxicology of acetaminophen.*

Acetaminophen is metabolized partly to a toxic metabolite called NAPQI. Under normal circumstances, NAPQI is detoxified by glutathione, and there is no toxicity. However, in overdose situation, glutathione is quickly depleted, NAPQI accumulates, and causes hepatic necrosis. N-acetylcysteine can replenish glutathione and act as an antidote.

982. *Discuss the toxicology of salicylates.*

Salicylates initially stimulate respiration, causing an increase in body pH. With time, there is muscle fatigue, leading to acidosis. Salicylates also directly interfere with ATP production which contributes to the acidosis. Seizures, hyperthermia, cerebral edema, pulmonary edema and cardiac arrest will eventually occur. Treatment consists of sodium bicarbonate and dialysis.

983. *Discuss the toxicology of tricyclics antidepressants.*

Tricyclic antidepressants are not prescribed much anymore, because newer classes have less toxicity. The three categories of toxic effects from tricyclic antidepressants are anticholinergic, alpha-blocking, and inhibition of fast sodium channels. Clinically these effects are manifested principally as tachycardia, hypotension, seizures, and cardiac arrhythmias. Sodium bicarbonate can be used as an antidote.

984. *Name a drug class that can be toxic if consumed after its expiration date.*

Tetracyclines can decompose over time to a metabolite that is toxic to the proximal tubule of the kidney (Fanconi Syndrome)

985. Name the most common over-the-counter drug seen in overdose situations and their symptoms.

Acetaminophen-liver necrosis
Non-steroidal anti-inflammatory drugs-gastrointestinal bleeding
Diphenhydramine-seizures, hallucinations, anticholinergic symptoms
Dextromethorphan-seizures, respiratory distress

ALCOHOL AND DRUG ABUSE TOXICOLOGY

986. *Name some drugs that cause hallucinations by interacting with serotonin receptors.*

Lysergic acid diethylamide (LSD)
Mescaline
Psilocybin
Peyote

987. *A person was involved in a car accident at 1 AM, and a blood alcohol level (BAL) is done at 4 AM which is 30 mg/dL. Assuming complete absorption at 1 AM and an elimination rate of 18 mg/dL/ hour, what was their level at the time of the accident.*

BAL @ 1 AM = (time difference x elimination rate) + BAL @ 4 AM.

$$= [\,(4 - 1) \times 18\} + 30$$
$$= \quad 54 \quad + \quad 30$$
$$= 84 \text{ mg/dL or } 0.084\,\%$$

988. *How does naloxone work in opiate overdose.*

Naloxone is a pure opiate receptor antagonist. It binds to the opiate receptor, but does not have agonist activity. In overdose situations, it competes with opiate agonists like heroin at the receptor. It knocks many opiate molecules off the receptor, lessening the overall effect of heroin.

989. *Explain why blood cocaine levels fall in an unrefrigerated body after death.*

Unlike like most drugs, cocaine can be metabolized by enzymes in the blood. After death, these enzymes can still be very active for some time if the body temperature is not lowered to decrease the metabolic activity. In a body at room temperature for several days, most of the original cocaine would be metabolized, and the blood cocaine level would be falsely low, compared to the actual level present at the time of death.

990. *Explain why chronic marijuana users may have significant blood tetrahydrocannabinol (THC) concentrations for days after cessation of smoking.*

THC is very fat soluble and builds up in the adipose tissue of chronic users. These fat stores are slowly released back into the blood during the period immediate post smoking cessation.

FORENSIC AND ANALYTICAL TOXICOLOGY

991. *Explain why fentanyl is considered a potent opioid, but does not turn the standard urine drug screen for opiates positive.*

The standard urine drug screen for opiates reacts to drugs that contain the opiate nucleus (heroin, morphine, codeine, hydromorphone). Although fentanyl binds to the opioid receptor, it is structurally dissimilar to naturally occurring opiates, and will not react in the urine test that is specific for the opiate nucleus. To detect fentanyl and other opioids without the opiate nucleus, special tests are needed.

992. *What is chain of custody?*

As applied to forensic toxicology, chain of custody is the documentation of the of the events from acquiring forensic evidence, to reporting analytical results by a certified forensic laboratory.

993. *Name some alternative biological materials that can be used for illicit drug testing.*

Hair, nails, saliva, vitreous humor (postmortem)

994. *When is the method of standard additions used?*

If there is no control matrix available (like in the analysis of exhumed liver), different amounts of test drug are added to a constant amount of analysis samples. An analysis of a data plot of instrument signal versus concentration will reveal the analyte concentration.

RADIATION TOXICOLOGY

995. *Describe the mechanism by which radiation damages DNA.*

Ionizing radiation interacts with matter by forming a positively charged atom and an electron. It may directly ionize an atom within DNA, or it may ionize other atoms near DNA such as oxygen and form free radicals which damage DNA by an indirect effect.

996. Define linear energy transfer (LET) and give example of low LET and high LET radiation.

LET is the energy lost or transferred to another atom per unit distance traveled. X-rays, beta particles, and gamma rays produce few ionizations per unit length and are considered low LET. Neutrons and alpha particles transfer large amounts of energy per unit length and are considered high LET.

RISK ASSESSMENT

997. Define margin of safety.

Margin of safety is a parameter that assesses the relative safety of a drug in a population. It is the ratio of the toxic dose to 1 % of the population to the effective dose in 99 % of the population.

Margin of safety = TD01/ED99

TOXICOLOGY IN THE FUTURE

998. What is proteomics?

Proteomics is an attempt to measure the types and amounts of all proteins made by a cell. In the future, it may be possible to correlate a form of protein expression with a specific toxic response.

999. What is metabolomics?

Like proteomics, metabolomics is an attempt to measure amounts and types of small molecules that occur in response to, diet, environment, disease, or toxicant.

1000. *What is systems toxicology?*

A recent definition is "the integration of classical toxicology with quantitative analysis of large networks of molecular and functional changes occurring across multiple levels of biological organizations".

References

Most of the questions in this book came from the following excellent toxicology textbooks.

Casarett & Doull's Toxicology: The Basic Science of Poisons. 8th ed., ed. C. D. Klaassen, (New York: McGraw-Hill, 2013)

U.A. Boelsterli, Mechanistic Toxicology, 2nd ed, (Boca Raton: Taylor & Francis Group, 2007)

K. E. Stine and T.M. Brown, Principles of Toxicology. 3rd ed., (Boca Raton: Taylor & Francis Group, 2015)

F.C. Lu and S. Kacew, Lu's Basic Toxicology, Fundamentals, Target Organs, Risk Assessment, 5th ed., (New York, Informa, 2009)

E. Hodgson, A Textbook of Modern Toxicology, 4th ed., (Hoboken, New Jersey, John Wiley and Sons. 2010)

S. Howard, Drugs of abuse: Pharmacology and molecular mechanisms, 1st ed., (John Wiley and Sons. 2014)

M. H. Dong, An introduction to environmental toxicology, 3rd ed., (Create Space Publishing. 2014)

J. Ladou. Current occupational and environmental medicine, 4th ed., (McGraw-Hill. 2007)

About the Author

D r. Richard Fruncillo spent most of his professional career as a clinical pharmacologist/human toxicologist conducting phase 1 clinical research studies for a major US pharmaceutical Corporation. In addition to being a practicing internal medicine physician, he has an undergraduate degree in chemistry and a PhD in biochemical pharmacology. He is certified by the American Board of Internal Medicine, the American Board of Clinical Pharmacology, and the American Board of Toxicology. He has previously taught pharmacology/toxicology at the medical/graduate school level, and is the author of many scientific publications in the areas of basic and clinical pharmacology/toxicology. Currently, he is a consultant to the medical and legal professions in the areas of pharmacology, toxicology, and drug development.

www.ingramcontent.com/pod-product-compliance
Lightning Source LLC
Chambersburg PA
CBHW051624170526
45167CB00001B/52